Weight Loss:

Ins and Outs

2013 Edition

by

Neil Ibrahim, MD

I0438779

Ibrahim University Foundation

120 Dr. Ibrahim Ln.

Summertown, TN 38483-5198, USA

Copyright ©2014 by Neil Ibrahim, MD

All rights reserved, including the right of reproduction in whole or in part in any form.

Weight Loss: Ins and Outs

Printed In the United States of America ISB 13-978-1494472627

Dedication

To

Very special people in my life:

Mrs. A. Odom, my LCHS Algebra teacher;

John Beasley, DDS, and Mike Bailey my baseball coaches;

Jeff Valentine, my Boy Scout Master;

My brothers at Sigma Nu Fraternity at GW; and last but not the least to

My mom, Carolyn Glover, MS; my dad, Monier Ibrahim,

PhD; my brother, Dean Ibrahim, MD; and my always gracious aunt Faye Glover for their constant encouragement and unconditional love.

"Writing a book is a horrible, exhausting struggle, like a long bout of some painful illness. One would never undertake such a thing if only was not driven on by some demon that one can never resist nor understand."

George Orwell, 1946

Disclaimer

This book contains the experiences, ideas and opinions of the author. It is only intended to provide helpful and informative material on the science and art of dieting. Neither the author (the copyright holder) nor the publisher is engaged in rendering medical, health, or any other kind of personal services in this book. Seek medical advice for your ailments from your own physician. Medical treatment (by surgery or medications) in America is not delivered except to human patients <u>in person</u> by a federally and state licensed physician to practice medicine in America.

The author, copyright holder, and the publisher specifically disclaim all responsibility for any liability, loss, or risk, personal or otherwise, which is incurred as a consequence, directly or indirectly, of the use and application of any of the contents of this book.

This book was funded partially by

Ibrahim University Foundation

- For a better world®

Other books by Neil Ibrahim, MD

All these books are in paperback and eBooks and found at www.bookfinder4u.com

1) ACT with Writing Option

2) SAT II in Math IIC, Biology E/M, Chemistry & Writing

Table of Contents

PART I

A Ticking Time Bomb

Foreword

Chapter 1

A Ticking Time Bomb

"While it's often daunting to take risks, it's even scarier to not be able to mold to the changes that life throws at you. Don't wait for the mere chance that greatness will find you. Go out there and demand it."

Catherine O'Connor, BS, GW class of '07

During the Capitol Commencement of

The George Washington University

Foreword

"No passion so effectually robs the mind of all its powers of acting and reasoning as fear." Edmund Burke

I was enrolled at the Little League baseball despite my young age of 9 at the six grade because the players for the Little League were chosen according to their school grades- not their age. I should have been in Babe Ruth baseball. What an intelligent young boy, Neil, in classroom gain at the dugout of Bobby Brewer Baseball field, Lawrenceburg, Tennessee? I gained nothing except anger and stress because I wanted my excellence in classroom to be matched on Bobby Brewer Baseball Field. Parents tried to calm the young Neil, but they failed because I did everything possible to stay away from the dugout; lots of ego or will. At one midnight I was sneaking at our Frigidaire for my ruts of several scoops of ice cream and multiple slices of home-made desserts, which were prepared by the award-winning Mom in cooking from her early teens. And my dad said, "Do you know that an Indian lady survived stranded on the Himalayas for ten days without food and research shows that rats die from over-eating?" I sarcastically told Dad that I am not stranded on the Himalayas and definitely I am not a rat." Dad ruefully said," You are missing the point." Of course, I know my dad's point that I am killing myself by overeating, but I had no better choices.

After the baseball season was over, I got enrolled in the Boy Scouts of America where I had time to relax, sell cookies and other merchandises to raise funds for BSA camps, and enjoy myself. Several weeks later, Mom asked me to help her in cooking some delicious recipes of my choice. Within a month, I began to sleep better, gain self-esteem and lose weight. Most of all, throughout our choice of recipes for menus, I began to understand what is a healthful ingredient and what is not to include in a healthful diet.

My calamity opened my eyes to many of my friends' and other people's waist size and their bodies' shape; is it an apple or a pear shape? With time, research, and experience, I began to accumulate the wisdom and discover the flaws of other diet books. Either they are asking too much in too little time; promising too much more than they can deliver; asking people to live on energy; forgetting the human nature of committing mistakes; providing supplemental recipes; providing unbalanced diets; turning people to carnivores; or making people more paranoid about food.

In this book, you will find the wisdom and experience of more than 200 dieters, their families, and friends with what works and what does not work. Read this book carefully and take notes before you advance into the recipes' section. There is no way to follow a recipe unless you understand the reason behind adding or removing that ingredient from that diet. This book is written to accommodate different levels of understanding of science, and I added a layman's glossary to close that gap. Neither you nor your healthcare provider has the time or probably the knowledge to research the subject carefully. I do not expect you to understand every word in this book, but I do expect you to have a broad understanding of the subject at hand.

Pharmaceutical companies send sales agents to inform your physician about new drugs and bombard the airways constantly with their advertisements; I am an impartial voice for you and your physician to make a wise decision. Always bear in mind, if a 9- year- old Neil can do it, you can do it too. Happily, thanks God, I am a dapper, honor medical student, and alumni award recipient of The George Washington University, Washington, D.C.

Happy dieting,

Neil Ibrahim, MD

Food & Cooking Diagnostic Test

What do you really know about cooking and food? Let's see.

1) *Which activity consumes the most of your life time?*

a. Breastfeeding and changing diapers.   B. Cooking

b. Eating and digestion.   d. Foreplay and sex.

2) *Which oil fits oven-heated cooked meals at high temperature, 400⁰ F?*

A. Extra-virgin oil.   b. Sesame oil. c. Canola oil. d. Sunflower oil.

3) *Where do you find cholesterol?*

a. Plants. B. Animals   c. Mushrooms.   d. None.

4) *Which choice is true?*

a. All fats are oils.   b. Cholesterols are fats.

c. Fat in chicken is marbled in meat.

d. Dark meat has more calories than breast meat of poultry.

5) *Which meal has shown to level insulin levels?*

a. Peanut butter and oat bran bread.   b. Honey with cereal.

c. Corn syrup and pancake.   d. Chocolate with ice cream.

6) *Which choice is recommended to cut your food appetite?*

a. Milk chocolate. b. Soda. c. Oat bran bread.   d. Crackers.

7) *Which organ (s) is (are) the most responsible for food digestion?*

a. Heart. b. Liver.   c. Stomach.   d. Kidneys.

8) *Which method is the least effective to lose weight?*

a. Smoking nicotine. b. Sex.   c. Starvation.   d. Smoking marijuana.

9) *Which spice has shown to help in weight loss?*

a. Oregano.   b. Rosemary.   c. Red pepper.   d. Cinnamon.

10) *Which diet is the most effective in weight loss?*

a. Eating fat-rich foods.   b. Eating only two large meals every day.

c. Eating frequently small meals.   d. Eating carbohydrate-rich meals.

11) *What does your body crave for under extreme stress?*

a. Hot sex.   b. Sweet food.   c. Dark chocolate.   d. Budweiser beer.

12) *Which country has the highest percentage of obese people?*

a. Mexico.   b. India.   c.USA.   d. Italy.

13) *Which food has the most calories for equal amount of food?*

a. Fiber.   b. Syrup.   c. Soda.   d. Fat.

14) *What is the healthy BMI for a woman?*

a.14   b. 24   c. 34   d. 44

15) *Which vitamin is the most likely to be destroyed by cold storage?*

a. C   b. D   c. A   d. K

16) *Which environment would most likely to encourage food gorging?*

a. Eating with a partner.   b. Eating alone in bright lights and TV.

c. Eating alone with classical music. d. Eating in small plates.

17) *Which physical activity is the most effective psychologically and physically in weight loss?*

a. Stretching. b. Stationary cycling.   c. Indoor exercise. d. Walking.

18) *Which number has the most adverse effects in your health?*

a. Bra size. b. Blood pressure. c. Blood sugar level. d. Breathing rate.

19) *Which vitamin is **not** manufactured by your gut flora?*

a. A   b. B   c. Folic Acid   d. K

20) *Which food etiquette is effective for weight loss?*

a. Drinking before eating.   b. Finishing up your plate.

c. Conversing during eating.   d. Eating before a hot sex.

Food & Cooking Diagnostic Test

Cryptogram of Answers

1. 79	6. 164	11. 69	16. 104
2. 118	7. 73	12. 108	17. 153
3. 77	8. 112	13. 157	18. 62
4. 166	9. 161	14. 66	19. 171
5. 185	10.180	15. 175	20. 100

You do not have to be a CIA or a KGB agent to crack this cryptogram; the other way is to read the book to find the answers.

Green, unroasted coffee beans

30 g fiber/day

Eat Tuna fish, banana &turkey to sleep

No junk foods with additives

No food 4 hours before bedtime

No insomnia

No stress

No diseases for obesity	low fiber food intake
No genes for obesity	lots of junk foods
No supplements	snacking before bedtime
No high sodium or sugar foods	stressful life style
No more than 30% from carb foods	gene/ disease that causes obesity
Breast feed while child	pickles/ sweeteners/ supplements
No loud noises during sleeping	processed foods
No snoring	more than 30% of carbohydrates
No sleep apnea	non –breast feed while child
No hypertension	sleep apnea/snoring
No diabetes	diabetes/hypertension
Sleep in dark or red light	sleep in white or blue lights
8 hours of sleep daily	shift work or neighbor's dog bark
Exercise ½ hour daily	sedative life style
1500-1800 calories/day	2000 or more calories daily

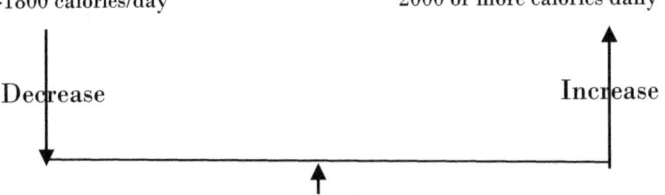

Decrease   Increase

A Typical See-Saw of Body Weight

A TICKING TIME BOMB

"100 % American and 37 % Obese,"

George Bernard Shaw, revised

Notwithstanding my revised version is not thrilling, it made me feel better than the original version. The original version is "100% American and 99% stupid."

Well, our, USA, calculation of obesity is different from the World Health Organization's (WHO) calculations because WHO's calculation is much lenient than our calculations.

Obesity because of poor nutrition and lack of exercise is a "ticking time bomb" for life expectancy levels. The World Health Organization (WHO) defines obesity and overweight as an accumulation of excess body fat to an extent that may impair health. Excess fat is measured as the body mass index (BMI), where a person weight (in kilograms) is divided by the square of his or her height (in meters). WHO defines overweight as a BMI of 25 or more and obesity as a BMI of /or more than 30. Body-builders and pregnant women are not included in this definition. For example, a person of 5' 6" person of height and 160 pounds of weight will be,

5' 6" = 66 inches x 2.54 (centimeters per inch) / 100 = 1.68 meters.

160 pounds= 160 x 0.373 (kilogram per pound) = 59.68 kilogram.

BMI = Weight / (Height x height) = 59.68 / (1.68 x 1.68) = **21.4.**

In our (USA) calculation of obesity:

BMI= Weight (Pounds) x 703 / (height (inches)^2 .

5' 6" = 66 inches   with 160 pounds (weight), BMI will be,

BMI= 160 x 703 / (66)^2 = **25.82.**

How have you measured up? Well, you are not alone; actually obesity is a worldwide epidemic. Of course, we (USA) are number # 2 in the number of overweight people with 34%; Mexico 37%; UK 23%; Canada 14 %;Turkey 12%; Germany and Spain 13%; Sweden and Denmark 10%; France, Austria and Italy 9%; and Japan and Korea 3%, but there is a silver lining lately that 19 states reported a 1% decrease in obesity rates and 10% decrease in obesity in K-12 kids according to 2013 CDC reports. No wonder that obesity in the United States costs $51.7 billion annually, 5.7 % of health care dollars, $90 billion in future expenses and $30 billion on time lost while away from the market place. Obese people are not happy either about their bodies; they view their bodies as loathsome or grotesque. Obesity is a national security problem in the United States because 30 percent of military volunteers are turned down because of their obesity and $12 billion dollars are lost in productivity in the job because of obesity. Further, obesity is the number one risk factor for six types of cancers such as pancreatic, esophageal, colon, kidney, prostate and breast cancer.

One might ask, "Why do I need to lose weight for?"Although beauty is on the eyes of the beholder, slimness has many advantages:

1) Slim people have better chances of getting better jobs, dates, sex lives (slim men have higher libido than their overweight counterpart men- obese women and men have higher estrogen than testosterone and lower testosterone levels decrease libido in men);

2) Better longevity- football players have an average age of 51;

3) Less healthcare costs and cheaper insurance (overweight people pay 20- 40% higher insurance premiums than their slim counterparts); in addition, 51% of Americans' health insurance premiums are paid by their employers and those insurance premiums are tax-deductible as business expenses. In other words, your health problems are taxed at tax-payers' expense. Fact: only 17% of

Americans are business owners and the rest are employees -despite loose claim of capitalists.

4) Less chance of snoring and better REM sleep and less chance of sleep apnea, heart diseases, stroke, acid reflex, and fatigue. Obese people are deprived of the most important part of sleep that is the slow sleep, when consolidation of information is processed in the brain during the slow sleep, and therefore, they develop Alzheimer's disease at a young age.

5) Less chance of getting vehicle accidents- obese people have as much nine times of getting vehicle accidents as their slim counterparts;

6) Less chances of getting divorce or cheat on their spouses;

7) Obese parents are less inclined to engage in social and athletic activities with their children and most likely to have obese children because of their lack of physical activity, poor nutrition, or just their genetic disposition to be obese.

8) If all of the above did not convince you to lose weight, here are the scary ones: a) 18% of mortality rates in USA are due to obesity; b) every ten percent of body weight you lose increases your life span by 2 years; c) obese people pay more money in airlines, insurance, clothe, and in lost of opportunity in life e.g. marriage, employment, income, social activity, etc.; and d) obese people experience migraine headaches as much three times as non-obese individuals.

Ten of the 14 states with the highest percentages of obese people are in the Southeastern of USA. Truck drivers with BMI of 28 (overweight) are required by the federal law to submit to a sleep test to assure their adequate sleep and less involvement in truck accidents on the roads (the average cost of a truck accident is $3.1 million in comparison to $70,000 for a car).

Are you the one to blame? Not exactly, your parents bear thirty percent of the blame because they made the batter that is missing some good genes and the rest are environmental factors under your control. Hallelujah, your body weight is under your control. Seventy percent of your body's cholesterol is made by your body and thirty percent is from diet intake. Although $40 billion are spent annually by weight loss seekers, there are many hurdles. The slim figures of the Pharaohs, the Vikings, and other ancient, legendary people, reveal that obesity's rise coincided with:

(1) Modern food processing such as puffing, mechanical and thermal treatments, and cutting of whole grain that leads to a rupture of the granule, exposing the individual starch molecules for enzymatic activity. Consequently, the digested starch molecules are absorbed rapidly through the walls of the small intestine, and insulin levels are elevated higher than the same amount of a more slowly absorbed carbohydrate with a low glycemic index such as a whole grain or rye. This modern food processing is cheaper than the conventional stone-ground process, and the flour has a much longer life in storage. However, it removes the embryo and seed coat (bran), whose fiber impeded the milling process;

(2) Dwindling of free-range birds (chicken, ducks, and geese) and fish- farming of salmon, trout, sturgeon, catfish, and tilapia eliminated the essential long- chain omega- 3 fatty acids, which modulate metabolism;

(3) Widespread of saturated and hydrogenated fatty acids because they oxidize (become rancid) less than unsaturated fatty acids, which has a short shelf-life;

(4) Decrease physical activity because of the need for automobiles because of zoning ordinances, far-away work places, television, video games, and personal computers. Further, gang violence and row housing are two major impediments for physical activity in inner cities;

(5) Introduction of corn is a major factor. Obesity in the Pima Indians in the southwestern United States increased by 50 % after their utilization of corn, a large-kernel crop; that was substituted for the traditional small- kernel, fibrous ears of maize;

(6) Invention of corn syrup has taken the market by storm. Corn syrup is made from cornstarch by boiling it with acid under pressure and a highly concentrated sugar- fructose- is obtained. This high-fructose corn syrup, whose sweetness matches that of sucrose (table sugar), is cheaper than sugar obtained from sugar cane or sugar beet. Manufacturers put immense quantities of it into soft drinks, ketchup, ice cream, juice, and many other food products; and

(7) Finally pro-lobbying by the processed food and Cola manufactures, sugar cane growers, and the packed- food industry has been influencing our governmental policies.

Women are more prone to obesity than men for several factors: (a) women are more sedentary than men; (b) women snack more than men; (c) women diet more than men, so their bodies resist diets; (d) women are frequently on hormone supplements, of their own or replacement, which make it more difficult to lose weight and may cause them to gain weight; (e) women may exercise less vigorously and have less muscle mass to burn energy sources less than men; (f) women tend to participate more in aerobic exercises, while men jog or use highly resistant exercise machines; (g) women snack more than either working women or men, who are away from home most of the day; (h) birth control pills (progesterone) increase appetite and promote fat storage. However, estrogen increases insulin sensitivity and weight loss. The most common oral contraceptives" the pill" contain a higher concentration of a progestin (similar to progesterone) and a lower concentration of estrogens; (i) women are genetically more efficient in fat storage because their bodies are designed to support two people rather than one; and finally, (j) repetition of pregnancy among some women without having enough intervals between giving birth and pregnancy.

Am I asking you to return to chewing the fibrous sugar cane, hunting animals, and gathering honeycombs and nuts as our ancestors did for eons? Of course, it is too late. However, take charge of your health because unfortunately, even your physician may not be able to help you for many factual reasons:

only 34% of patients disclose to their physician adverse effects of obesity as sleep apnea. And men are known for bad-mouthing sleep.

There is a silver lining in this book because I will arm you and others with the knowledge needed to have a healthy and long life; lose weight and keep it; enjoy your favorite food without deprivation or guilt; and most of all answer the most frequent questions in your mind. You wouldn't dare to ignore a valuable advice from The George Washington University alum and MD. Would you?

Project

Most grocery stores have scales; therefore, while shopping at your favorite grocery store, weigh yourself and calculate your BMI. Record your BMI at your weekly journal and compare your results with BMI calculations in chapter 12.

PART II

The Anatomy of Food

"But faith, fanatic faith, once wedded fast to some dear falsehood, hugs it to the last."

Thomas More, Poet

Chapter 2

Carbohydrates

"Potatoes are for pigs and corn is for cattle."

A popular French adage

Carbohydrates are chemically made up of carbon, hydrogen and oxygen, arranged in ring structures. The simplest carbohydrates are made up of single- ring sugars; glucose, fructose (fruit sugar), and galactose (milk sugar), collectively called monosaccharide. Disaccharides are made up of two ring structures linked together, such as maltose (two glucose molecules), produced by sprouting grains and the main sugar in beer. Sugar-cane and sugar-beet plants make sucrose- a disaccharide- or table sugar. Lactose (milk sugar) is also a disaccharide of glucose and galactose rings linked together. In some people, especially senior citizens, the mucosal cells of the small intestine fail to produce enough lactase, the enzyme necessary for digestion of lactose. This deficiency results in a condition called lactose intolerance- common among eastern Jews. Undigested lactose retains fluid, and bacterial fermentation of lactose results in the production of gases. The major symptoms of lactose intolerance are diarrhea, flatulence, bloating, and abdominal cramps after consumption of milk and other dairy products.

The third category of carbohydrates is called polysaccharides; these large carbohydrates are composed of many monosaccharide linked together. They include glycogen (mainly stored form of carbohydrate in humans in the liver and skeletal muscles), starch (main carbohydrate in food), and cellulose (main carbohydrate form in plant leaves and stems) - not digested by humans but adds bulk that aids movement of food through intestines. Like disaccharides, polysaccharides can be broken down into monosaccharide. For example, when the blood glucose (sugar) level falls, liver cells have the ability to break down glycogen into glucose and release it into the bloodstream. In this way glucose is made available to body cells.

Glucose molecules draw water toward them; this property makes it impossible for plants and humans (animals) to store energy in the form of glucose because too much storage of glucose would quickly swell and burst the cell. Therefore, plants often turn glucose into starches that do not swell and burst cell and are convenient for storage of energy for later use. The most common storage sites for starch are roots (sweet potatoes), underground stems (white potatoes), fruits (winter squashes), and seeds (beans and grains). When we eat starchy vegetables, fruits, and grains, our body turns these complex carbohydrates (amylose and amylopectin) back into glucose for metabolic fuel.

Carbohydrates are mostly found in grains; here is a comprehensive list of the food content of carbohydrate rich foods.

This section includes food contents (Calorie (cal), carbohydrate (carb), fat, protein (prot), and fiber) in grams; cholesterol (chol) and sodium (sod), in milligrams (mg) for all fresh and raw foods. I do not want to include canned and processed foods because they change according to manufacturers and they are usually included on food labels. Please compare only foods listed in similar measures. This is usually confusing between measures by capacity and measures by weight. I included a table in the appendix for making such conversions.

Please bear in mind that seasonal and regional differences affect the nutritional content of most foods.

A) Grain- based foods (no cholesterol in all plant -driven foods)

Food	Cal	prot	carb	fat	Sod	fiber
Bagel (4 oz)	270	10	18	1.0	620	4
Barley flour (1/4 cup)	93	3	19	0.5	0	3
Black bean (1/3 cup)	120	8	20	0	240	11
Bread - bran(1 slice)	120	5	20	2	220	2
Broad- bean (1/2 cup)	40	3	6	0.4	28	23

Food						
Buckwheat-flour (1cup)	100	4	21	1	0	3
Carob flour (1 cup)	425	5	92	1	36	41
Corn -fresh (5 oz)	123	5	27	2	21	4
Corn-flour (1 cup)	422	8	90	5	6	16
Couscous-dry (1/4 cup)	210	7	43	0	5	3
Croissant -plain (1 pc)	290	4	30	17	340	0
Cowpeas (1/3 cup)	130	8	21	0	250	11
Garbanzo-dry (1/4cup)	170	10	29	2	10	6
Hummus (1/2 cup)	160	7	13	9	180	3
Kaput flour (1/4 cup)	110	4	25	0.5	0	4
Kidney beans, dry (1/4 cup)	160	11	29	0	0	10
Lentil-dry (1/4 cup)	70	8	19	0	5	9
Lima beans (1/2 cup)	88	5	16	1	6	4
Macaroni -whole wheat(1 cup)	174	8	38	1	4	4
Millet flour (1/4 cup)	110	4	26	1	0	2
Navy bean-dry (1 oz)	100	6	17	1	0	8
Noodle (1 cup)	210	8	43	5	400	2
Oat flour (1/3 cup)	120	5	20	2	0	4
Pasta -plain (2 oz)	211	7	43	1	4	2
Pinto beans-dry (1/4 cup)	150	10	27	1	0	8
Rice -dry (1/4 cup)	150	4	33	1	0	1
Sorghum-whole grain (1cup)	650	28	143	6	12	3
Soy flour (1/2 cup)	200	16	16	9	0	8
Soybean-shelled (draw)	188	17	14	9	19	6
Tabouli (1/2 cup)	160	5	30	4	210	5
Tofu -fresh (1/2 cup)	94	10	3	6	9	2
Waffle, 1 pc	140	3	19	5	300	1
Wheat-flour (1/4 cup)	100	4	22	0	0	3
Wild rice, raw (1/4 cup)	170	6	35	0	0	2

The difference between the structural characteristics in carbohydrates affects the speed of their conversion into glucose. This difference is a major determinant of the glycemic-index, of how fast various starchy foods affect our blood sugar levels.

Which in turn, affects our energy, our tendency to gain weight, and of course our general health. In general, high glycemic-index foods stimulate strong insulin responses, increasing exposure of the body to all the harmful effects of insulin. On the other hand, low glycemic -index foods do not imbalance insulin levels because they provide energy in a slow, sustained-release form, mitigating hunger and facilitating the smooth use and storage of calories.

The following factors affect the glycemic -index (GI) of foods.

a) The physical structure of food: Breads have high GI because the fine particle size of wheat flour gives digestive enzymes great surface area to work on, and the exploded structure of bread, a result of the leavening action of yeast, further increases the surface area for digestive enzymes action. However, *al dente* pasta that Italians favor resists digestive enzymes more than longer-cooked pasta and so has a lower GI.

b)The puffing process: Rice cakes and crisp bread have high GI because the starch in rice is puffed up, offering a great surface area for digestion, whereas sugar (sucrose) has a low GI.

c) The presence of fiber: Fibrous coats around beans and seeds and the cellulose in intact plants restrict access of digestive enzymes to the starch within. The fiber in whole wheat is insoluble, but cracking and milling remove the physical barrier (fiber or bran) and make starch (flour) more accessible to digestive enzymes.

d) The presence of fat: Fat presence in food reduces the GI by slowing the rate of emptying of the stomach and the digestion of starch too.

Glycemic index measures how fast different carbohydrate foods affect blood glucose. The higher the GI, the faster is the rate of increase of glucose in the blood, the higher the insulin levels, and the greater of potential of the toxic effects of high blood sugars. I want to make two points to illustrate the difference between the Calorie content and GI:

1) Glycemic index is totally different from Calorie content because all carbohydrates have the same Calorie value from the same amount of carbohydrates; one gram of potato or fructose gives off 4 Calories. In other words, although one gram of fructose has a GI of 23 and one gram of potato has a GI of 95, both fructose and potato (carbohydrates) give off 4 Calories per gram consumed.

2) A lot of people confuse GI with Calorie content; therefore, I will give you some examples to clarify my point.

Example

Almond (House of Bazzini), 1 ounce, gives off 170 Calories, and has 6 grams of protein, 6 grams of carbohydrate, 14 grams of fat, and 2 grams of fiber. In this case, its carbohydrate content is 6/30= 20% of the total content; that is why nuts (almond included) have a low GI of 15- 30.

Example

Oat bran (dried), 1 ounce, gives off 70 Calories, and has 5 grams of protein, 19 grams of carbohydrate, 2 grams of fat, and 4 grams of fiber. In this case, the carbohydrate content is 19/ 28.4 (ounce) = 65%. That is why oat has a GI of 50-65.

The Glycemic Index of Some Popular Foods

Low GI foods: below 45, intermediate: 45-65, and high GI: more than 65

a) Grain Based Foods

High GI

White bread and French bread	95	instant rice	90
White pretzels	85	Rice cakes and rice Crispies	80
Corn, corn chips, Graham		Croissant, Corn meal, White	
Crackers, regular crackers, white		rice, Taco shells, cream of	
Bagel, Total cereal, Cheerios,		wheat, Shredded wheat- white,	
Puffed wheat, and Cornflakes	75	Melba toast, and Millet	70

Intermediate GI

Grape Nuts, Whole-Wheat Crackers,		Pita bread- regular,	
Nutri-grain cereal, Stoned Wheat Thins,		Rye sourdough,	
And Regular pasta--------------------65		Wild rice, brown rice,	
		Oatmeal, special K, and	
Buckwheat grouts, popcorn--------55		Muesli- no sugar added ----55	
Whole-grain, cracked wheat,		Sponge cake, pita bread-	
Bulgur bread, whole rice,		stone ground, wheat grain,	
Oat and bran wheat----------------50		Barley grain, whole grain	
Noodles -instant	45	pasta, All bran -no sugar—45	

Low GI

Rye grain	35

b) Vegetables and Fruits

High GI

Dates, dried-------------------------103		Broad beans-----------	79
Baked potatoes, parsnips----	95	Rutabaga--------------	72
Red -skinned potatoes--------------88		Beets------------------	69
Sweet corn, sweet potato, banana- 54		Cantaloupe, pineapple 65	
Carrots, yam, and kiwi-------------	50	Baked beans, peas	48

Mango, papaya----------------------55   Grape, orange---------- 45

Plantain banana--------------------- 45   Ripe banana------------ 60

Raisins-------------------------------- 65

Low GI

Navy beans, apple, pear, plum   38   Kidney beans, grapefruit 28

Chickpeas, fresh peach, Mulkhia   Watermelon --------------- 7

Dried apricot, lentils--------------- 31   Cherries, soybean----------22

Lima beans, olives--------------------30   Pinto beans--------------- 40

Soy beans, peanuts, tomatoes ---- 15   Nuts---------------------- -20

c) Dairy foods

Milk

   ---Whole   22   Ice cream -----------------------60

   ---Skim   32   low fat------------------- -------- 50

   --Chocolate flavored-------43   Yogurt, low fat----------------33

d) Beverages

High GI

Gatorade™-----------------------------78   Fanta™----------------68

Intermediate GI

Flavored Syrup (diluted)------------- -66   Orange juice----------46

Low GI   Apple Juice --------------   40

e) Candies

High GI

Jelly beans ----------------------80   Life Savers™, Skittle Fruit Chews-70

Intermediate

Chocolate -------------------- -49

Low GI

Snickers----------------------- 41   Twix Cookie Bar----------------------44

f) Sugars -High GI

Glucose --------------------- 100   Maltose (in beer)---------------- 105

Sucrose (table sugar)--------- 65

Intermediate GI

Honey------------------------ -58   Lactose-----------------------------46

Low GI: Fructose(in grape & honey)- --------------------------------- ------23

Unfortunately, the glycemic index is not available on the labels of nutrient contents. Reading labels is essential and most contents are listed in the order of their abundance.

Project

Classify the foods in your pantry and refrigerator according to their GI values, and record your results at the weekly journal.

Chapter 3

FAT

"Any who act as if freedom's defenses are to be found in suppression and suspicion and fear confess a doctrine that is alien to America."

Dwight Eisenhower

Fats (lipids), like carbohydrates, may be utilized to produce energy. Each gram of fat produces about 9 Calories, about twice that of carbohydrates and proteins. If the body has no immediate use to them, they are stored in fat depots throughout the body and in the liver. Lipids are used in transport of cholesterol, blood clotting, and myelin sheaths around neurons to speed up nerve conduction. Cholesterol, another lipid, is used in the synthesis of bile salts, steroid hormones (e.g., cortisol), and sex hormones (estrogen mostly in females and testosterone mostly in males).

Lipids include fats, oils, fatty acids, and compounds derived from them. Fats are very common in milk and products, nuts and seeds. The following is the food content of all fat-rich foods.

d) Nut and seed based foods

Food	Cal	prot	carb	fat	sod	fiber
Almond shelled (1/2 cup)	360	12	12	30	0	8
Cashew-halves (1/2 cup)	340	12	14	28	0	2
Flax seeds (1/2 cup)	190	7	15	13	0	9
Filbert chopped (1/2 cup)	312	7	9	36	0	3
Macadamia-shelled (1/2 cup)	480	5	9	51	1	3
Peanut shelled (1/2 cup)	428	17	15	36	4	6
Pilli shelled (1/2 cup)	430	6	3	48	2	2
Safflower-dried (1/2 cup)	288	9	20	41	1	2
Sesame whole (1/2 cup)	400	14	16	40	4	10
Sunflower dried (1/2 cup)	330	11	14	28	2	6
Walnut shelled (1/2 cup)	420	10	6	40	0	6

e) Milk- based foods (in 8 fl.oz)

Food	Cal	prot	carb	fat	chol	sod
Cow whole	150	8	12	8	35	270
Cow 2%	130	8	12	5	20	125
Cow 1%	110	8	12	2.5	10	125
Goat -fresh	168	9	11	10	28	122
Human	171	3	17	11	32	42
Sheep	264	15	13	17	66	108

Most fatty acids in our body are hooked together onto glycerol. Glycerol is a simple compound of carbon, hydrogen, and oxygen derived from the breakdown of glucose. When three fatty acid chains are linked into a glycerol molecule, triglycerides are formed. Most fats stored or transported through the bloodstream in our body are in the form of triglycerides. Bile from the liver, which is stored in the gallbladder, plays a major role in digestion of fats. Triglycerides also comprise the main fat in food, accounting for 95 % of the fat we eat. Stored triglycerides in our body's fat depots are primarily reserves of energy (calories).To free those calories, our body separates primarily saturated fatty acids (SFAs) and monounsaturated fatty acids (MUSFAs) from glycerol for energy use. Stored glycerides are also reserves of essential fatty acids (EFAs), and Polyunsaturated fatty acids (PUSFAs) which are reserved for critically important regulatory roles in our body.

Saturated fatty acids and partially hydrogenated fatty acids are usually solid at room temperature 25^0 C (77^0 F) because their melting points are higher than unsaturated fatty acids (MUSFAs and PUNSFAs) melting points. Some of these saturated fatty acids' melting points are shown: Lauric 44^0 C, myristic 59^0 C, palmatic 64^0 C, and stearic 74^0 C. Saturated fatty acids are very common in animal fat, butter fat, coconut oil, palm kernel oil, and palm oil. Unsaturated fatty acids (MUSFAs and PUSFAs) are mostly liquid at room temperature; some of these unsaturated fatty acids' melting points are shown: Oleic 4^0 C, linoleic -5^0 C and linolenic -11^0 C. MUSFAs are very common in olive oil (77%), canola oil (62%), peanut oil (49%), and avocado oil. PUSFAs are very common in fish oil, flaxseed oil (72%), cottonseed oil, grape seed oil, safflower oil, sesame oil, soybean oil, sunflower oil, walnut oil, and corn oil. Saturated fatty acids raise LDL (bad cholesterol) and decrease HDL (good cholesterol). Values of lower than 110 (mg/ dl) for LDL and higher than 35 (mg/dl) for HDL are healthy.

Because unsaturated fatty acids become rancid (oxidized) relatively quickly, manufacturers began to "hydrogenate" them; a process that makes them more stable with long- shelf life. Unfortunately, during the hydrogenation process, *trans* fatty acids are formed. It takes a bit of more energy to introduce the hydrogen into an unsaturated fatty acid (oleic) backbone in the *cis* position than in the *trans* position. Therefore, almost all saturated positions of the backbone assume the more stable form- the *trans* form. Moreover, the trans- form is unlikely to switch into the *cis*- form. These *trans* fatty acids increase LDL cholesterol levels and reduce HDL cholesterol levels. In other words, *trans* fatty acids are detrimental to cardiac health. *Trans* fatty acids are very common in margarines (the more solid the margarine, the more the trans fatty acids; stick margarines contain the most, tub margarines contain less, and the semi-liquid margarines contain the least). Avoid high-fat baked foods, such as doughnuts, cookies and cakes, and any product for which the label says, "partially hydrogenated vegetable oils." Luckily, all natural MUSFAs and PUSFAs are *cis*-fatty acids.

The other class of fatty acids is called essential fatty acids because they are not synthesized in humans. Plants and animals are capable of synthesizing saturated fatty acids first from glucose. Both are also capable of synthesizing MUSFAs and PUSFAs after-words. However, only plants are capable of introducing unsaturated points (double bonds at 3 or 6 positions) early in the chain in the fatty acids' backbone; thus making omega -3 and omega 6- fatty acids. Animals can put un-saturation points farther down the backbone but not up front as plants do; they lack the enzymes to do so. Yet humans need both omega-3 and omega-6 fatty acids for important functions and even die without them. That is why linolenic (omega-3) and linoleic (omega-6) fatty acids are essential.

No wonder, why we buy our eggs from the Amish? Amish's chickens are free-range chicken. Although chicken (animals) are not capable of making omega-3 fatty acids any more than we, they can eat them from plant life and store them in the yolk of their eggs. In fish farming of salmon and sardines, the omega-3 content of foods derived from them is determined by their diet. Chicken, salmon and sardines in the wild get their omega-3 by eating algae and other simple forms of plant life. Some American markets have fortified eggs, one high in omega-3 fatty acids. Egg farmers get that omega-3 fatty acid - rich eggs by fortifying chicken feed with a meal made from algae. Lack of omega-3 fatty acids (linolenic) is marked by skin inflammation, increased susceptibility to infection, growth retardation, and eventually death. Luckily, all these symptoms, except death of course, are reversible if linolenic acid is restored to the diet. Omega-6 fatty acids' deficiency leads to growth retardation, lack of coordination, and impairment of learning ability. Essential fatty acids are the starting materials for the synthesis of a very important class of hormones, prostaglandins. Prostaglandins govern many aspects of basic life especially the healing process, blood clotting, and immune function. Interestingly, prostaglandins derived from omega-6 fatty acids promote inflammation and blood clotting, while prostaglandins derived from omega-3 fatty acids oppose those effects. Omega-3 fatty acids are available from plant sources such as flaxseed, hemp seeds, soybean, and walnuts as well as animal sources such as fish, herring, mackerel, salmon, and sardines. Omega-6 fatty acids are available from plant sources such as cottonseed oil, grape seed oil, peanut oil, safflower oil, sesame oil, soybean oil, corn oil, and sunflower oil as well as animal sources such as meat and poultry. I want to make three crucial points regarding essential fatty acids:

1) If the fatty acid is omega-3, it is capable of introducing other un-saturation points down the backbone. For example, EPA (eicosapentaenoic acids), very prevalent in salmon and sardines,

and DHA in fish oil can be made from linolenic acid (omega-3 rich). However, our body cannot make them if it lacks the starting material (omega-3 fatty acids).

2) The ratio of omega -3 to omega-6 in the diet is very crucial because too many omega-6 fatty acids inhibit synthesis of EPA or DHA. Too many omega-6 fatty acids compete for the same limited supply of enzymes and decrease omega-3 fatty acid synthesis.

3)Beef fat (0% linolenic, 2% linoleic), lard fat (0% linolenic, 10% linoleic), Olive oil (2% linolenic, 5% linoleic), canola oil (7% linolenic, 30% linoleic), and linseed oil (52% linolenic, 20% linoleic). From the previous analysis, lard and beef fats are devoid of omega-3 fatty acids, and the richest source of omega- 3 fatty acids is linseed oil, followed by canola oil. That explains the preference for canola oil to olive oil in our pantry.

Some people claim that canola oil has up to 5% erucic acid, a toxic fatty acid, but this toxicity is mitigated by the extraction process.

Hemp (*Cannabis sativa*), source of marijuana, is a well known plant throughout the world as a source of a delicious, greenish, nutty flavor, and essential fatty acid-rich oil. Although growing hemp plants is illegal in America (except Colorado and other Northwestern states), hemp oil is available in natural food stores.

Project

Poor small amount of canola oil, olive oil, and clarified butter in separate open containers and let them sit. Each day, sniff the containers and record when you detect the odor of rancidity in each at your journal. Hint: Heat and light will enhance rancidity.

Project

Classify the oils and fats in your pantry and refrigerator into SFA, MUSFA, and PUSFA. Record your classification at your journal.

Chapter 4

Protein

"Tell me what you eat, and I will tell you what you are,"

Jean Brillat-Savarin- 19ᵗʰ - century food philosopher

During our volunteer work at the Boy Scouts of America, in my early teens: Pick -up Garbage Day of very old people and Cleanup Day at Davy Crockett Park, my dad usually said," You can tell a lot about people [wealth, education, health, beliefs, age, etc.] from their own garbage."

Wheat has gluten (protein). Since wheat grains are smaller than corn grains, during the stone-grinding process, lots of seed coats (bran) remain in wheat flour than in corn flour. A 1/4 cup of wheat (Mills) gives off 160 Calories, and has 6 grams of proteins, 34 grams of carbohydrates, 1 gram of fat, and 7 grams of fiber, but a 1/4 cup of corn (Mills) gives off 120 Calories, and has 5 grams of protein, 24 grams of carbohydrates, 1 gram of fat, and most of all 4 grams of fiber.

One day, I asked a vegetarian, "Where do you get your omega-3 fatty acids and essential amino acids in your diet?" He elegantly replied, "You might ask the billion people whose diets have been vegetarian for millennia." Walter Mondale in his presidential campaign in 1984 said, "Where is the beef?" Mondale campaign's slogan reflects historical, cultural, and economic attitudes toward protein consumption. Actually, research has confirmed the validity of vegetarian diets. Our body is clever enough to scavenge the essential amino acids from the 10^{14} bacteria that inhibit the lower intestinal tract, worn - out red blood cells, or from the vast numbers of cells that slough off the lining of the digestive tract every day, or the omega-3 fatty acids supply. I elaborated earlier that free-range animals get theirs from plants originally. Actually, human's protein needs are much lower than most people think, and the risk of protein deficiency for most of us is negligible. We basically need 1 gram of protein for every kilogram of body weight; 1/1000 of our weight is our daily requirement of protein. In other words, a

160- pound person (70 kilograms) needs 70 grams of protein daily. Proteins are mostly found in meats and seafood. The following is the food content of the protein-rich foods.

f) Meat - based foods (in 4 ounces)

Food	Cal	prot	carb	fat	chol	sod
Beef (braise, lean)	274	34	0	15	105	79
Chicken dark meat only	232	31	0	11	105	105
Chicken light meat only	196	35	0	5	96	87
Ham meat only	239	33	0	11	107	73

g) Seafoods (in 4 ounces)

Food	Cal	prot	carb	fat	chol	sod
Caviar	300	38	3.6	17	20	250
Clam-raw (meat only)	84	15	3	1	39	64
Cod raw (meat only)	93	20	0	1	49	62
Crab raw (meat only)	95	21	0	1	47	448
Fish raw	104	21	0	2	54	92
halibut raw	124	24	0	3	37	61
Herring raw	180	21	0	10	68	102
Lobster raw	102	21	1	1	108	0
Ocean perch raw	102	21	0	2	48	85
Octopus raw	93	17	3	1	54	261
Oyster raw	93	11	6	3	0	120
Salmon raw	207	23	0	12	67	66
Shrimp raw	120	23	1	8	173	168
Tuna raw	163	26	0	6	43	44

Unlike carbohydrates and triglycerides, which are stored, proteins are not warehoused for future use. During digestion, proteins are broken down into their constituent amino acids; each gram produces about 4 Calories. These amino acids may be used to produce energy or synthesize new proteins for body growth and repair. Excess dietary amino acids are not excreted in the urine or feces but rather converted into glucose (gluconeogenesis) or triglycerides (lipogenesis). Liver cells, convert amino acids to fatty acids, ketone bodies, or glucose. Ammonia, a by-product and toxic substance of protein metabolism, is converted to urea by the liver cells. The kidneys eliminate urea from the bloodstream and excrete it in the urine. Proteins provide our body's needs of non-essential amino acids. Of the 20 amino acids in our body, 10 are called essential amino acids. We are unable to synthesize eight (lysine, methionine, leucine, isoleucine, phenylalanine, threonine, tryptophan, and valine) and synthesize two others in inadequate amounts, especially during childhood (arginine and histidine). These essential amino acids are synthesized by plants or bacteria, and foods containing these essential amino acids must be supplied for a healthy diet.

What are the pitfalls of a carnivorous diet? Increase workload on the liver and kidneys and possible exposure of sensitive organs (brain) of toxic metabolic waste such as ketones and ammonia are the major consequences of my protein -rich diets. Moreover, rise in ammonia levels causes loss of consciousness and eventually death. Actually, protein -rich diets have deleterious effects on liver and kidney patients. Increase production of urea in a protein-rich meal not only taxes the kidneys, it **requires diuresis**- an increase of water loss in urine- to flush urea out into urine. Women in sub-Saharan Africa have very strong bodies, although they eat grain-based diets and a small fraction of calcium. In contrast, Inuit people, who eat huge amounts of animal protein along with their fat, suffer severe osteoporosis because of limited exposure to sunlight especially in winter months. Vitamin D, a necessary vitamin for absorption and utilization of calcium, made from cholesterol upon exposure to sunlight. Casein, a protein in cow's milk, triggers allergic reactions in infants and young children. Exposure of children to casein too early- before the age of two- exposes children to asthma, eczema, allergy development, and possibly juvenile diabetes.

Animal protein sources include meat from buffalos, cows, pigs, goats, sheep, poultry, fish, and shellfish and from wild animals like deer, elk, antelope, and moose. Plant protein sources include mainly legume plants (beans and clover) and nuts. Animal and plant protein sources are equivalent in their energy output (4 Calories per gram of protein). Poultry differs from the meat of the large grazing animals in many ways:

1) Its fat is external to muscle instead of being distributed thought it; therefore, it is much easier to remove before cooking. This is an excellent way to cut down the deleterious effects of saturated fatty acids' consumption in fat.

2) Chicken fat has only 30 % of saturated fatty acids, and essential fatty acids especially in the free- range chicken. Egg and milk (animal proteins) are good sources of omega-3 fatty acids if they came from free-range animals. Goat and sheep milk is mainly used to make cheese, but goat's milk is most often recommended as a substitute for cow's milk for children, who are allergic or intolerant of cow's milk protein (casein). Goats' milk is somewhat closer to humans' milk in its composition. Senior citizens and eastern Jews are allergic to milk products because they lack the enzymes necessary to digest dairy products.

Cows' (5.5% fat) and buffalos' milk (7.5% fat) contain much more fat than human milk; fat in whole milk is found in ice cream, cheese and of course butter. Notwithstanding some people love the mouth feel and flavor of butterfat; butterfat is a natural source of trans- fatty acids. These trans-fatty acids, formed as a result of the bacterial transformation of unsaturated fatty acids in the stomachs of cows, are responsible for the high rates of cardiovascular diseases in our societies.

Fish is no longer the "poor man's meat" because of the awareness of the health benefits of eating fish and dwindling of fish populations around the world that jacked up prices. Saltwater fish species spend more time in coastal waters where contaminated effluents are affluent. Fish farming has its own problems because farmers routinely give antibiotics; furthermore, unless the feed is fortified to provide omega-3 fatty acids, farmed fish's nutritional value is less than of their wild counterparts.

Shellfish meats come from two different animals: crustaceans and mollusks. Crustaceans include crabs, lobsters, shrimp, and crayfish; they provide high -quality protein with little cholesterol content especially the non-farmed species. Mollusks: clams, mussels, oysters, and scallops; squid and octopus are also included in this category.

Plant proteins occur mostly in the seeds of the pod-bearing plants (legumes) such as beans, lentils and peas, and in small amounts in leaves and tubers of some plants. All these plants contain carbohydrates as well but with low glycemic index, and a few- soybeans especially- contain significant amount of fat. Soybeans are high in fiber and some vitamins like folic acid- a B complex vitamin. Although legumes are major components of the vegan diet, they require long cooking time to make them palatable and digestible. Further, they contain resistant carbohydrates that cause flatulence and other digestive problems. Soybeans, on the other hand, are rich in omega-3 fatty acids, proteins and phyto-chemicals, such as *iso*-flavones. Soybeans are a major staple for East Asians; they enjoy them hot or cold; those dishes are products of organically -grown soybeans without the toxic residues of pesticides' use. Proteins also are rich in some non-legume seeds such as sesame, sunflower and nuts (almonds, hazelnuts, walnuts), but they have too much fat to be useful as primary protein sources.

Celiac disease results in mal-absorption by the intestine due to the ingestion of gluten. Gluten is the water-insoluble protein fraction of wheat, rye, and oats. In susceptible persons, ingestion of gluten induces digestive disturbances. The remedy is to eat a diet that excludes all cereal grains except rice and corn.

Vegetable proteins are better than animal proteins in several ways; they are cheaper, less perishable, more fibrous, and lower in saturated fatty acids. Mushrooms are another source of dietary protein; they are neither animals nor plants. Frank owns The Peoples' Mushroom Co., in the Hippies farm, Summertown, Tennessee and offers the most delicious mushrooms in the world. Mushrooms offer important health benefits, such as enhancement of the immune system, reduction of serum cholesterol, and some protection from cancer. If you forage for wild mushrooms, do not eat raw mushrooms because they contain toxins that cooking destroys; be aware of rattle snakes too because they might be around!

Project

Search for the source of egg, milk, fish, shellfish, poultry, and meat in your refrigerator. Are they from farmed or free-range animals?

Project

Classify protein- foods in your pantry and refrigerator according to their saturated fatty acids content.

Chapter 5

Micronutrients

"Error of opinion may be tolerated where reason is left free to combat it."

Thomas Jefferson

Did you know?

* Stripping bran during the process of making white flour removes 80% of flour's magnesium.

* Vitamin C is heat labile; destroyed by heat, and cold storage removes up to 50% of tangerines' vitamin C. Asparagus stored for just one week can lose 90% of its vitamin C.

* Processing of meats removes 50- 70% of vitamin B$_6$ and freezing meats destroys 50% of B vitamins.

* Fresh salads and cut vegetables and fruits lose 40-50% of their value if they sit for more than 3 hours.

Our body needs much smaller amounts of micronutrients (vitamins and minerals) than the previously mentioned macronutrients fats, proteins and carbohydrates. Our body requires a few millionths of a gram a day of each of vitamins and minerals.

VITAMINS

Vitamins are necessary for health and growth and their deficiency causes certain sickness, impairment of body's defense, and possibly death. Vitamins fall into two categories: those that are water-soluble (B complex and C) and those that are fat-soluble (A, D, E, and K). Overdoses of water-soluble vitamins are not as harmful as fat-soluble vitamins because the excess is flushed out, but overdoses of fat-soluble vitamins carry harmful effects.

Vitamin C acts as a reducing agent that regulates metabolic reactions and constitutes a corner-stone of our body's defense system against the deleterious effects of oxidative stress. Vitamin C is rapidly destroyed by heat and is abundant in some vegetables and ripe fruits especially kiwi, elderberry, blueberry, citrus fruits, red peppers, and potatoes. It promotes protein metabolism, especially laying down of collagen in connective tissues. As a coenzyme, vitamin C may combine with poisons, rendering them harmless until excreted, works with antibiotics, promote wound healing, and scavenges oxidative particles. Deficiency of vitamin C causes scurvy (a disease marked by swollen gums, loosened teeth, and bleeding under skin), poor wound healing, and anemia. Mega doses of vitamin C, through supplements, cause kidney stones and scurvy when withdrawn.

B- Complex vitamins include: B_1 (thiamin), B_2 (riboflavin), Niacin (nicotinamide) B_6 (pyridoxine), B_{12} (cyanocoblamin), pantothenic acid, Folic acid (folate, folacin), and Biotin.

B_1 (thiamin) is rapidly destroyed by heat and excessive intake is eliminated in urine. It is found in whole-grain products, eggs, pork, nuts, and yeast. It is essential in carbohydrate metabolism. Deficiency of B_1 includes,

a) Beriberi: Partial paralysis of the smooth muscles of the digestive tract and atrophy of the skeletal muscles; atrophy of limbs.

b) Polyneuritis due to degeneration of myelin sheaths, impaired reflexes, impaired sense of touch, and poor appetite.

B_2 (riboflavin) is not stored in large amounts in tissues and excessive amounts are excreted in urine. Small amounts supplied by bacteria of the digestive tract and its dietary sources include yeast, beef, veal, lamb, eggs, whole-grain products, asparagus, peas, beets, and peanuts. It is involved in protein and carbohydrate metabolism. Deficiency of B_2 includes improper utilization of oxygen resulting in blurred vision, cataracts, and corneal ulceration. Dermatitis and cracking of skin may also occur.

B_{12} (cyano-coblamin) is **not** found in vegetables and is the only vitamin containing cobalt. It is found in milk, eggs, cheese, and meat. This vitamin is important in red blood cell formation, and amino acid synthesis. Pernicious anemia is a common disease of B_{12} deficiency (memory loss, weakness, mood changes, and abnormal sensation); also impaired osteoblast activity.

Niacin (nicotinamide) is found in yeast, meats, fish, whole-grain products, peas, beans, and nuts. Its function includes cholesterol metabolism, inhibition of cholesterol production and assistance in triglycerides breakdown. This is the same niacin prescribed by health-care providers for treatment of high LDL (cholesterol) and triglycerides. Principal deficiency of niacin includes pellagra, characterized by diarrhea, and psychological disturbances.

Folic acid (folate, folacin) is synthesized by bacteria of the digestive tract and found in green leafy vegetables; the name comes from foliage. Folic acid is essential in production of white and red blood cells. This is very important especially to pregnant women because its deficiency results in neural tube defects in babies born to folic acid-deficient mothers.

Other B -complex vitamins like B_6, pantothenic acid and biotin are produced by bacteria of the digestive tract and mostly found in whole-grain products, yeast and vegetables. Deficiency of B_6 and B_{12} are precursors in accumulation of high levels of homocysteine, a toxic amino acid formed in the metabolic breakdown of proteins, especially animal proteins. A high level of homocysteine is a risk factor for arterial disease, heart attacks, and may elevate the risk of cancer and other degenerative diseases.

Fat- soluble vitamins (A, D, E, and K) require bile salts and some dietary fat for adequate absorption.

Vitamin A is stored in the liver and found in carotene (in carrots), yellow and green vegetables and milk. Its function includes formation of photo pigments in the eye, and growth of bones and teeth. Deficiency of vitamin A results in dry skin and hair, increased incidence of ear, sinus, respiratory, urinary and digestive infections, and inability to gain weight.

Night blindness or decreased ability for dark adaptation is another problem associated with vitamin A deficiency. Overdoses of vitamin A cause menstrual irregularities, fatigue, and liver damage.

Vitamin D is synthesized from cholesterol upon exposure to sunlight and is found in fish oils, egg yolk, and fortified milk. Research has showed that 15-20 minutes of sunlight exposure, without sunscreens, are quite enough for the human body to synthesize the needed amount of vitamin D. This vitamin is essential for absorption and utilization of calcium and phosphorus from the digestive tract. Its deficiency includes rickets in children and osteoporosis in adults because of lack of calcium in bones. Deficiency of vitamin D is also a contributing factor for osteoporosis in the elderly, and is more likely to occur in people living at northern latitudes in the winter months and those who are shut in. Women are at risk of osteoporosis because of the decline in sex hormones much earlier in life than men. Overdoses of vitamin D cause kidney stones, hypertension, and high cholesterol.

Vitamin E (tocopherols) is stored in liver, fat tissues, and muscles. Its dietary sources include fresh nuts, wheat- grain, seed oils, and green leafy vegetables such as broccoli. This vitamin acts as antioxidants to inactivate free radicals, reduces scar formation, and acts as a natural blood thinner to reduce the risk of heart attacks. Vitamin E deficiency causes muscular dystrophy in monkeys and sterility in rats, and quite rare except in cases of people with liver disease, who are unable to absorb the vitamin from the intestinal tract. Overdoses of vitamin E result in breast tenderness and slow wound healing in humans. Supplements of synthetic vitamin E are usually a mixture of d and L -isomers, only d- isomers are active.

Vitamin K is produced by the intestinal bacteria and stored in the liver and spleen. Dietary sources include spinach, cauliflower, and cabbage. Deficiency of vitamin K causes delayed clotting time and excessive bleeding. People with risk of blood clotting are usually given anticoagulants clogs, blood thinners, like warfarin (Coumadin). Overdoses of vitamin K- eating of too much of vitamin K rich vegetables or consuming too much of green tea- undo the action of blood thinners and cause blood clotting.

Hyper-vitaminosis refers to an excess intake of one or more vitamins. High doses of certain vitamins are sometimes deadly. Rarely is vitamin overdose is the result of eating foods; rather, it usually stems from consumption of supplements e.g. bear liver supposedly contains enough vitamin A to kill a person.

MINERALS

There are twenty-eight naturally occurring essential minerals in our body; eating more fruit and green vegetables satisfies our body's requirement for most of them. Special situations that may warrant special attention to ingestion of adequate amounts of minerals include, iron for women who have excessive menstrual bleeding; iron and calcium for women who are pregnant or breast -feeding; and calcium for the elderly adults and northern latitude residents.

66% of iron in our body is found in hemoglobin of blood and the remainder is in skeletal muscles, liver and spleen. Normal losses of iron occur by shedding of hair and in sweat, urine, bile and blood lost during menstruation. Dietary sources of iron are meat, shellfish, egg yolk, beans, legumes, dried fruits, nuts and cereals. Large amounts of stored iron are associated with an increased risk of cancer. (Old iron plumbing pipes and cooking in old iron-skillets are the major sources of iron overdoses.)

Iodine is necessary for synthesis of thyroid hormones, which regulate metabolic rate, and excess amounts are excreted in urine. Dietary sources of iodine are seafood, iodized salt, and vegetables and fruits grown in iodine- rich soils.

99% of calcium in our body is stored in bone and teeth, and the remainder is in muscles and blood plasma. Absorption of calcium occurs only in presence of vitamin D. Excess calcium- in absence of vitamin D- is excreted in feces and small amount in urine. Dietary sources are milk, egg yolk, shellfish, and green leafy vegetables. Calcium is very important in formation of bones and teeth, blood clotting, normal muscle and nerve activity, glycogen metabolism, and synthesis of neurotransmitters.

Chromium is found in high amounts in brewer's yeast, wine, and some brands of beer. It's needed for the proper use of dietary sugars and other carbohydrates by optimizing the production and effects of insulin. Chromium helps increase blood levels of HDL (good cholesterol), while decreasing levels of LDL (bad cholesterol). Deficiency of chromium is rare, except in adult-onset diabetes (type II diabetes).

Sodium is usually taken in adequate amounts as sodium chloride- table salt- and eliminated in sweat and urine. Healthy people have no worry about sodium deficiency, but only those who exercise vigorously in hot environment and do not replenish the salt lost through perspiration. They can become weak, faint, and disoriented as a result of excessive sodium loss.

Overdoses of minerals are dangerous; for example, calcium mega doses cause drowsiness, extreme lethargy, and kidney stones. Zinc mega doses cause difficulty in walking, hand tremor, and involuntary laughter. Cobalt mega doses cause goiter and heart damage. And finally, selenium mega doses cause nausea, vomiting, fatigue, irritability, and loss of fingernails and toenails.

FIBER

Fiber, also known as roughage, is the indigestible part of food that makes up much of the bulk of the stool. Even though not a source of calories, vitamins or minerals contribute to our overall health. Fiber deficiency is a significant problem in our western diet. Dietary fiber consists of indigestible plant substances, such as cellulose, lignin and pectin, found in fruits, vegetables, grains and beans. Fibers may be classified as insoluble (resistant carbohydrate), which do not dissolve in water and soluble fibers, which dissolve in water. Insoluble fiber passes through the digestive tract largely unchanged and speeds up the passage of rest of the material through the digestive tract. Soluble fiber, on the other hand, is found in abundance in beans, oats, barley, broccoli, prunes, apples and citrus fruits. It has the consistency of a gel and tends to slow the passage of the material through the digestive tract.

Fiber-rich diets may reduce risk of developing obesity, diabetes, atherosclerosis, gallstones, hemorrhoids, **diverticulitis**, appendicitis, and colon cancer. Soluble fiber may help lower blood cholesterol level. One possible explanation for the relationship of soluble fiber to cholesterol level is that the fiber binds bile salts and prevents their re-absorption. Because cholesterol is a precursor to bile salts synthesis, it leads to use of more cholesterol to replace the bile salts lost by the binding action of soluble fibers.

Amount of 30 - 40 grams of fiber is recommended daily for optimum health; about twice what most western diets have. The easiest way is to eat lots of the seeded- fruits such as raspberries, blueberries, kiwis, prickly bear fruits, and grapes. For example, one cup of fresh raspberry (Dole) contains 8 grams of fiber; one cup of fresh blueberry contains 4 grams of fiber; one cup of sliced cactus pads contains 4 grams of fiber; and finally, one cup of fresh kiwi (Dole) contains 8 grams of fiber. Your health is worth eating cereals containing bran.

Eating lots of insoluble fibers causes flatulence and bloating for the same reason that beans are gases producing. Bacteria in the gut attack and digest the complex carbohydrates, releasing methane gas in the process. Therefore to avoid these problems, introduce more fiber into your diet slowly to determine what the proper level is for you. Fiber-supplements, pills and other powders interfere with minerals absorption and impede bowel movements without drinking lots of water. Vitamins, minerals and fibers are mostly satisfied by eating fresh fruits and vegetables.

Project

Look up for the protein content in the foods you have in your pantry and refrigerator?

Project

Classify those foods according to their vitamins and minerals.

Chapter 6

Phytochemicals

"Impossible is just a big word thrown by small men and women who find it easier to live in a world they have given than to explore the power they have to change it. Impossible is not a fact. It's an opinion. Impossible is potential. Impossible is temporary. Impossible is nothing."

Adidas

Phytochemicals are a large group of compounds- some made in the body and others provided by the diet- that work together to scavenge free radicals and other harmful substances. These phytochemicals are not essential, in that their absence in the diet will not result in death or serious dysfunction. Nevertheless, they are very crucial to combat the constant exposure of our bodies to dangerous organisms and toxins.

Phytochemicals are prevalent in all plant foods especially those that are deep green, bright yellow, orange or red. Foods like tomatoes, oranges, broccolis, strawberries, and carrots are excellent sources of plant pigments such as polyphenols, chlorophyll, carotenoids, and bioflavonoid.

Green plants especially contain large amounts of **chlorophylls**, which are detoxifiers and possibly anti-cancer agents. Chlorella and blue-green algae, beet greens, Choy, collards, dandelion greens, kale, mustard greens, and nettles are rich in chlorophyll. Blue-green algae have been credited with immune-enhancing effects and stimulation of responses to tumors and microbes.

Orange, yellow and red-orange foods are rich in **carotenoids** such as beta-carotene, lutein, and lycopene. There are more than 600 carotenoids occur naturally, but carotenes are the most widely known. Carotenes offer protection against lung, colorectal, breast, uterine and prostate cancer, through destruction of oxygen -free radicals in lipids.

Anthocyanidins, complex falvonoids, are found in blue, purple or red color foods such as beets, blackberries, blueberries, cherries, colored grapes, and purple cabbage. Anthocyanidins promote collagen formation and help protect blood vessels from oxidative damage. Proanthocyanidins are the precursors of anthocyanindins and are composed of smaller units such as catechins and epicatechins that are most commonly found in apples and green tea.

Sulfur -containing compounds are present in a variety of colorful foods including the crucifer family, garlic and pineapple. These sulfur-containing compounds are effective because sulfur offers protection against cancer and chelates mercury out of the body. The crucifer family (cruciferous plants) - is any of the various plants of the family Cruciferae. Cruciferous vegetables - vegetables of the mustard family- especially mustard greens, various cabbages, broccoli, cauliflower, turnips, kale (kail), kohlrabi, Chinese cabbage, spinach mustard, gold of pleasure (false flax), shepherd's burse, radish, and cresses. The crucifers-family's phytochemicals bind carcinogens in the gastrointestinal tract.

The lily family includes garlic (*Allium sativum*) and onion (*Allium cepa*), both of which contain sulfur compounds such as diallyl disulphide and diallyl trisulfide- two of the active agents in garlic oil- and S-allyl cysteine- found in crushed garlic to inhibit tumor and enhance immune response. Garlic, onion, and shallot prevent cancer and inhibit progression of existing cancers   especially N- nitroso- induced cancers. N-Nitroso cancers are potent carcinogens formed within the intestine as a result of the bacterial degradation of nitrates and nitrites, two common water and food chemicals that are used in the processing of ham, sausages and other meat products. Sulfur-containing compounds such as bromelain are found in pineapples. U.S. and French research shows oral bromelain can reduce cancer in animals especially leukemia and lung-cancer.

Limonene is a bioflavonoid substance found in citrus rind that breaks down carcinogenic substances. Also quercitin is another anticancer agent. Lignan- found primarily in rye and flax- weakens estrogens'effect that reduces estrogen-related cancers such as breast cancer and prostate cancer.

Genistein in red clover diminishes the growth of new blood vessels in cancerous tissues. Lentian- in shiitake (*Lentinus edodes*) and reishi (*Ganoderma ludidum*) and maitake (*Grifolia frondosa*) mushrooms - has anti-cancer potency.

Kelp and seaweed are also anticancer agents because they are rich in mucilaginous alginates. Mucilage and gums, like fibers, swell in the intestine and absorb liquid as well as toxins and the heavy metals. Japanese studies show regular consumption of kelp reduces cancer risk. Cayenne pepper, ginger, rosemary, sage, thyme, and turmeric have anti-inflammatory, anti-cancer and antioxidant properties. Research suggests that cur cumin, the bright yellow flavonoid present in turmeric (*Curcuma longa*) roots, selectively inhibits inflammatory agents in response to injury and irritation, causes constriction of blood vessels, and inhibits tobacco smoke carcinogenicity.

Eat fresh fruits and vegetables and stay healthy. Five to eight servings of fruits and vegetables are recommended daily for optimum health. A serving of fruit is one medium-slice of watermelon, one-quarter cup of dried fruits, or six ounces (three-quarters of a cup) of fruit juice. A serving of vegetables is one-half cup of chopped raw vegetables or the same amount of cooked vegetables, one cup of leafy, raw vegetables, one medium potato, eight to ten medium -size carrot sticks, or eight ounces of vegetable juice. Be sure to wash fruits and vegetables thoroughly before eating. Peeling is enough to get rid of all pesticide residues from carrots, banana, squash, corn, potatoes and most waxed vegetables like cucumbers and apples.

Project

Categorize phytochemicals in your pantry's food and record the results at your weekly journal.

PART III

The Anatomy of Appetite

"They go on in strange paradox, decided only to be undecided, and resolved to be irresolute, adamant to be impotent. The era of procrastination, of half measures, of soothing and baffling expedients, of delays, is coming to a close. In its place, we are entering a period of consequences."

Winston S. Churchill

Chapter 7

The Devil Duo

"The good opinion of mankind, like the lever of Archimedes, with the given fulcrum, moves the world."

Thomas Jefferson

Did you know?

*One-third of end-stage kidney diseases is due to diabetes.

*Four out of five diabetic patients die from cardiovascular disease (heart attacks, stroke, or peripheral vascular disease) initiated by diabetes.

*Diabetes is the leading cause of amputations and blindness in the elderly.

You might ask, "What is the devil duo?" Insulin and glucagon are the devil duo because they are the maestro, chief, or the conductor of food metabolism. Insulin is a hormone manufactured and secreted by the beta cells of the pancreas, but **glucagon** (another hormone) is released from the alpha cells of the pancreas. The principal action of glucagon is to increase blood glucose level when it falls below normal (hypoglycemia). Insulin, on the other hand, helps adjust blood glucose level by decreasing the level if necessary. The level of blood glucose controls secretions of glucagon and insulin by the pancreatic cells. The human pancreas stores about two- hundred units of insulin and normal people secrete about twenty-five to thirty units of insulin daily. Insulin sweeps glucose, amino acids, and free fatty acids into cells for storage as fat and glycogen to be used later.

Glucagon prevents hypoglycemia (low blood sugar) by breaking down glycogen in the liver to form glucose and conversion of muscle protein to blood sugar (gluconeogenesis).

Gluconeogenesis can occur during periods of excessive exercise or long starvation. During the first day of starvation, glycogen in the liver is utilized, and muscle proteins are used

59

after-words. Glucagon secretion is stimulated by hypoglycemia, fasting, and ingestion of a protein- rich meal. Although humans can survive without glucagon as in the case of pancreas removal, they must have insulin to survive through their own secretions or insulin injections. However, insulin injections are not an efficient method in providing a continuous supply in exactly the right amount as done by their own pancreas. As a result, diabetics on insulin injections often experience wide swings in their blood sugar levels.

Although glucose is the major stimulus for insulin secretion, fructose (a sugar from fruits) and amino acids (proteins) from meats cause a significant insulin release only in the presence of the previously elevated blood sugar- as is the case in overweight individuals because of excessive stimulation of the pancreas through over-eating and development of insulin resistance.

Wide swings in insulin levels (too low or too high) make weight loss almost impossible. High levels of insulin promote storage of sugars as glycogen in both the liver and muscle, and prevent the breakdown of glycogen and triglycerides (fat). Insulin also promotes the storage of fat as triglycerides in fat cells and protein in muscle cells. Insulin further activates lipase (an enzyme) that speeds up the removal of triglycerides from the bloodstream and their deposits in fat cells. Moreover, insulin inhibits another lipase (lipoprotein lipase) that breaks down stored fat. The net effect of insulin on lipase enzymes is an increase in stored fat that results in weight gain and an increase of abdominal girth. To make matters worse, insulin facilitates conversion of blood sugars and amino acids (lipogenesis- through glyceraldehyde 3- phosphate) in the blood into fat. In short, insulin is a major deterrent to fat breakdown and major contributor of fat storage.

Obesity is the net effect of insulin and glucagon imbalance. In type II diabetes (non- insulin dependent diabetes), insulin resistance (a condition of decreased responsiveness to insulin), fat, liver and muscle cells have become insensitive to normal levels of circulating insulin. As a result, small bursts of insulin are not detected and more insulin is released. No wonder, why obese individuals with type II diabetes have elevated levels of circulating insulin, cholesterol, and blood sugar. Unfortunately, notwithstanding obese individuals may suffer only of elevated insulin levels with normal blood sugar- their pancreas finally becomes exhausted from the constant stimulation by glucose (sugar) and finally fails, resulting in developing diabetes.

Syndrome X is a combination of two or more of insulin resistance with resulting elevated insulin levels, elevated triglycerides, obesity, high blood pressure, and coronary artery disease. Insulin resistance is the precursor of the other symptoms of Syndrome X. This syndrome offers a great insight about insulin resistance; fifty percent or more of insulin resistance can be reduced or even reversed because insulin resistance is not a genetic trait. In other words, insulin resistance is treatable by less carbohydrate consumption, combined with exercise and cessation of smoking to reduce circulating insulin. Lowering circulating insulin levels and decreasing insulin resistance decrease obesity incidence and heart disease progression.

There are three categories of diabetics: Type I diabetes (insulin-dependent) are mostly younger, thinner and require regular daily injection of insulin because their pancreas does not make much insulin. Type II diabetics (non- insulin dependent) are generally older (over 40) obese, and can be treated with diet alone or diet and oral medications because their bodies do not respond to insulin. Type III diabetes (gestational diabetes) is mostly common in pregnant women. Although this type of diabetes is temporary, over time fifty to seventy percent of gestational diabetics develop type II diabetes, especially those who are obese before or after pregnancy. Untreated gestational diabetes has a major impact on the mother and her unborn child; therefore, screening for gestational diabetes is advised between the twenty-fourth and the twenty-eight weeks of pregnancy for all obese, pregnant women. Diabetes deteriorates vision, cardiovascular system, kidneys, and nervous system.

Ingestion of 50- 100 grams (200 - 400 Calories) of glucose during a high- sugar meal, raises insulin levels and keeps them elevated for several hours. Therefore, eating high-carbohydrates (e.g., high glycemic index foods) three times a day and bedtime snacks cause insulin elevation for eighteen out of the twenty-four hours. Whether you have central obesity (apple shape) or pear shape obesity (obese butt), ingestion of high glycemic foods (carbohydrates) and bedtime snacks are the major culprits. Apple shape obese individuals have beer bellies, and thinner hips and buttocks- most common in diabetics and insulin resistance. Pear shape obese individuals have their fat distributed in the hips and buttocks. Fortunately, Ingestion of low glycemic diets drops cholesterol levels by seven to fifteen percent after six weeks and insulin secretions by thirty -two percent after two weeks. Ingestion of a sugar-rich or high-glycemic, carbohydrate-rich meal initially causes the blood sugars to rise with an associated significant insulin spike. However, when the insulin finishes its work and blood sugars begin to fall, it often drops below normal, hypoglycemia (50 mg /dl in adults), and in low blood sugar. Normal blood sugar (glucose) is 90 to 110 milligrams per deciliter (mg/dl). Blood sugars below 40 mg /dl often require medical attention. Hypoglycemic persons are often lethargic and anxious. They usually want to eat something, usually another sugar- rich, carbohydrate-rich meal to elevate their blood sugars. This cycle between craving and ingestion of sugar-rich meals creates insulin resistance, obesity and diabetes.

I know that you are already tired of insulin and glucagon, but I had to guide you through this very important interplay of hormone actions. You are probably wondering, "What the heck is the glycemic index?" I will get to that in the next chapter, but I want you first do the next two projects for your own health and wellness.

Project

Look at your body after shower and decide whether you have an apple or pear obesity. Write down your obesity type in your weekly journal.

Project

Buy over- the counter blood sugar measurement kit or make a visit to your health-care provider, and record your blood glucose (sugar) level at your weekly journal.

Chapter 8

A Second Brain

"We must consider that we shall be a City upon a

Hill, the eyes of all people shall be upon us."

John Winthrop, A.D. 1639

All of us grew with the idea that our brain controls everything in our bodies; well, not precisely true. The hypothalamus (inside the brain) regulates your body temperature, feeling of rage, aggression, pain, body pleasure and behavioral patterns of sexual arousal. The hypothalamus also regulates food intake through two centers: the feeding (satiety) center is responsible for hunger sensations and the thirst center for producing the sensation of thirst.

The Satiety center is controlled by two counterbalancing chemicals; namely, CART and NPY.

1) CART increases metabolism, reduces appetite and increases insulin delivery to make more energy of food rather than be stored as fat; (Defense system).

2) NPY decreases metabolism and increases appetite; (Offense system).

It turned out that CART system is stimulated by another hormone, leptin, which is secreted by stored fat in your **omentum**. NPY, on the other hand, is stimulated by another hormone, ghrelin, which is produced in the intestine. When you are hungry or losing weight, your body cells become more sensitive and responsive to leptin action; leptin stimulates CART. However, when your stomach is empty, it releases ghrelin to make you want to eat by stimulating NPY.

Clues: Deprivation diets do not work because increased ghrelin secretion sends more signals to eat. Especially Ghrelin signals, short-term signals, send hunger signals twice an hour. But leptin signals are long-term signals. Clues: Keep level of leptin high enough to counterbalance the effect of ghrelin. How!

By eating satisfied food; there is no deprivation. Actually, your satiety center is waiting to be turned off by NPY or stimulated by CART. Whichever fills up the site first is what controls whether you want to eat more or not. After ingestion of a satiating meal, another hormone (CCK) is released from the intestine.CCK counterbalances the effect of ghrelin.

A handful of nuts turn off your desire to eat by inhibiting production of NPY or producing more CART. But eating simple sugars, fructose (fruit sugar-in beer, sweeteners, soft drinks, corn syrup, and salad dressing), and galactose (milk sugar) act as NPY suppressants and consequently you want to eat more.

Understanding how to increase leptin and decrease ghrelin is more important than learning about them. How could we increase leptin or decrease ghrelin?

1) **Avoid HFCS** (High Fructose Corn Syrup), simple sugars, and processed food because they are coated with fructose and simple sugars.

2) **Eat unsaturated fats** because saturated and *trans* fats produce low levels of leptin than unsaturated fats. Lesson: stay away from sausage, cookies, and whole-milk dairy products (saturated fats). Increase intake of: canola oil, sesame oil, and olive oil (unsaturated fats).

3) **Drink 2- 3 cups of water** to quench your thirst. Remember, thirst center is very close to appetite center. Clues may be your desire for food is not because of hunger rather than thirst. Lesson: when you feel hungry, try to drink a cup of water at first to see whether you are still hungry or you were just thirsty.

4) **Have sex:** actually, sex helps in many ways: a) To satisfy the satiety center because satisfying the sex center satisfies the appetite center. And (b) having sex will keep you occupied away from the fridge.

5) **Stay away from high glycemic- index carbohydrates** because they increase NPY, which makes you hungry. Translation: eat lots of low-index carbohydrates, fruits, and vegetables.

6) **Avoid alcohol binge:** Limit your intake of beer (mainly fructose sugar) to one medium size can a day. Red wine has protective effects on arteries, but limit your intake of wine to a half glass daily.

7) **Control your hormonal surge** by eating healthful foods such as nuts, fruits and vegetables.

8) **Live stress-free life:** Stress increases NPY and stimulates fat cells to grow in size and number. Actually, research has shown that intake of high-fat and high-sugar diets to stressed subjects increased the worst kind of obesity, the apple -shaped type, which makes people more susceptible to heart disease and diabetes. Stressed people deposit abdominal fat (omentum) 40% more than unstressed people. Make peace around yourself to decrease life stress: be kind and helpful to others because in turn you are surrounded by a peaceful life. Research shows that the main recipient of kindness and help to others is the helper himself rather than the one receiving the help because the helper gets more positive psychological, social, and physiological effects than the one receiving the help or kindness acts. Remember, laughing stimulates more muscles than crying.

Coping With Stress through Exercise:

a) **Breathing exercise:** Sit or lie down while your legs and arms are uncrossed. Take a deep breath and push out as much air as you can. Breathe in and out again, this time relaxing your muscles on purpose while breathing out. Keep breathing and relaxing for 5-10 minutes at a time. Do these exercises at least three times a day.

b) **Loosen- up exercises:** Circling, stretching, and shaking parts of your body. This exercise is better with your favorite motivating music.

c) **Change thoughts:** Each time you notice a bad thought, deliberately think of something that makes you happy or proud, memorize a poem, a prayer, or favorite quotes to replace bad thoughts.

d) **Reverse breathing exercise:** In this exercise you will exhale first and then inhale, do this while watching your body.

e) **Accept the problem:** by saying, " This problem isn't really so bad after all."

f) **Problem- solving attitude:** Some people say to themselves, "What can I do about this problem?" Then they try to solve the problem.

g) **Add positive to your life:** Starting an exercise program, joining a sports team, taking dance lessons or joining a dancing club, starting a new hobby or learning a new craft, and finally volunteering at a hospital or your favorite charity.

h) **Patch things up:** If you are at odds with a friend, a partner or a relative, you can make the first move to patch things up. Archbishop of South Africa and Nobel Laureate, Desmond Tutu, once said that the best way is to approach whoever offended you and tell him or her "I forgive you." The Archbishop's advice is very valuable because it puts an end to your unfavorable thoughts about this person and starts a new thought of friendship or at least a neutral relationship. In my early days of high school, I was bullied by a classmate because of my academic and athletic excellence before my teen years. When I told my dad, he said," Tomorrow ask this kid to join you at Boy Scouts of America or at the Baseball field." I did exactly what Dad said not because of my understanding of my dad's advice but of my exhaustion of this bully's acts. It turned out that this bully kid only needed a warm, accepting, welcoming environment that he lacks at home. He and I became buddies and he quit bullying me, as well as others in our school.

Chapter 9

Exercise Activity

"Give me a fish, and I will eat for a day.

Teach me to fish, and I will eat for a life time."

Old Chinese Proverb

*Research shows that individuals with daily physical activity for six months or more have six times as much recovery and improvement of heart diseases as non-physically active individuals.

*American Cancer Society research shows that 150 minutes of regular exercise, e.g. walking, weekly cuts the occurrences of breast cancer in postmenopausal women by 14%.

* Research shows sitting 11 hours or more increases cancer occurrences by 34%.

Why do you need to exercise to lose weight? First, the answer is simple, exercise burns calories and tips the scales in your favor for weight loss. For example, if you eat 2,000 calories and walk 2 miles (250 calories), you actually decreased your caloric intake into 2,000- 250= 1,750 calories. It is that simple; if you burn more calories than you eat, you will lose weight. Second, exercise helps in maintaining or building strong muscles. Third, exercise improves your mental well-being. Walking strengthens muscles, rejuvenates memories, improves social lives and metabolism, and empowers psychological well-being. Walking is the most powerful, easy, inexpensive body exercise for well-being

How much exercise do I need to lose weight? That depends on your health and your weight-loss goal.

Are you healthy enough to exercise? To answer that, read the following questions honestly, and circle the right answer.

Y/N Do you have a joint problem that could be made worse by physical activity?

Y/N Has your physician ever told you that you should only do physical activity under supervision?

Y/N Within the last four weeks, have you ever had chest pain during your physical activity?

Y/N   Are you under prescription drugs for heart or blood pressure problems?

Y/N Do you suffer of dizziness or loss of balance?

Y/N Do you ever lose consciousness upon standing?

Y/N Do you know of any other conditions that might be aggravated by physical exercise?

If you answered **NO** honestly to **all questions**, you can include physical activity as part of your weight-loss program. Your exercise program varies in frequency (the number of days per week); duration (the amount of time spent per session); and intensity (how hard do you exercise). My daily walk around our land – almost 2 miles- rejuvenates my energy and heightens my future outlook.

Exercise levels: Depend on **age** and exercise **level.**

a) **Beginner:** Whoever has not participated regularly in physical activity within the last six months, calculate your heart rate x 60%; for example,

a 50 -year -old person will be,

(220- 50 years of age) x 0.60 = 102 beats (pulses/ minute).

b) **Intermediate:** You currently exercise. Heart rate will be,

(220- 50 years of age) x 0.70 = 119 beats (pulses/ minute).

c) **High end:** You have been exercising for more than a year.

(220- 50 years of age) x 0.80= 136 beats (pulses/ minutes).

If you are a beginner, your current physical endurance cannot sustain physical activity much beyond 60% or 102 heart beats per minute. Take it easy and exercise within your Maximum Heart Rate (MHR): Beginner (60%), intermediate (70%) and high end (80%).

The following table shows a 15- week exercise plan:

Week	Frequency (sessions/week)	Intensity (% of MHR)	Duration (minutes/ session)
1	2- 3	60	15- 20
2- 5	3- 4	60- 70	20- 25
6- 10	3- 4	65- 75	25- 30
11- 15	3- 5	75- 80	30- 45

The following table contains energy expenditure for men (160 pounds); women's energy expenditure is usually about 80% of men's energy for comparable activity.

Physical Activity (50- 250 Calories/ hour)

Lying or Sleeping (80), Sitting (100), Softball game (100), Shopping at a yard sale (160), Desk Work (110), Driving (120), Fishing (130),   Standing (140), Housework (180),Washing your car (250), Mingling at a block party (140), Cheering at your child's softball game (100), Strawberry picking (200), and Throwing a Frisbee (100).

Physical Activity (more than 200 Calories/ hour)

Bicycling: 5.5mph (220), 11mph (440), 16.5 mph (660)

Boating: Canoeing- 2.5 mph (230), Row boat -2.5 mph (300)

Bowling (270), **Chopping Wood** (720), **Computer work:** (200)

Construction: (480); **Dance:** Slow Step (300), Square Dance (350), Aerobic -fast step dancing (490), **Fire-fighting:** (600)

Golf: Golf cart (150), walking (300), hunting (200- 300)

Jogging- 5 mph (640), 6 mph (750), 10 mph (1200), **Masseur** (480); **Nursing :** (350), **Playing with kids** (480)

Racquet Sports: Badminton (350), Racquetball singles (775), squash or handball (600), Tennis Singles (420), **Shoveling** (400),

Skating - 10 mph (400), **Skiing:** Cross Country Skiing (900), Downhill Skiing (600), Waterskiing (460), **and Swimming** 0.25 mph (300)

Walking (100), 2 mph (150), 4 mph (330), **Weight lifting** (vigorous) (720)

Yard Work: Gardening (220), Power Lawn Mower (250), and Watering plants (300)

Pulse Measurement

Your pulse (hear beat) is the strongest in the arteries closest to the heart. The pulse may be felt in any artery that lies near the surface of the body. The radial artery at the wrist is the most commonly used to feel the pulse. Resting pulse rate in a normal person is between 70 and 80 beats per minute.

Chapter 10

Shopping

"I would that God the gift would give us,

To see ourselves as others see us."

Robert Burns, Poet

I had to do a science project in the eighth grade, and my dad suggested finding the relationship between people's shopping habits in Super Wal-Mart and Kroger stores and their waist size. Here is what I found:

a) 75 % of adult obese people purchased items from the interior sections of the stores;

b) 90% of teenagers did their shopping in the interior sections of stores;

c) 90% of adult obese people purchased most of their items in the second or the third isles of the stores;

d) 80% of adult obese preferred whole milk to reduced fat milk;

e) 90% of adult obese people preferred white bread to wheat or 100% whole-grain bread;

f) 75% of adult obese people preferred Pepsi and Coke to diet brands; and

g) 60% of reduced (with coupons, discounts, or buy two for the price of one) items were Pepsi, Cola, Pizzas, and processed foods.

I need to mention that almost all supermarkets have their vegetables, fruits, meat, cheese, fish, and poultry in the periphery of the store. The interior sections usually have breads, grains, processed foods, Colas, Pepsi, Pizzas, and ice creams. Moreover, the first two to three sections of store are usually reserved for ice creams and pizzas. This opens my eyes to the effect of shopping on health at an early age. I earned an A in science, as I usually do, earned an Eagle Scout badge in community service for his project, and most of all I had a great time watching people's crazy habits of shopping at grocery stores without regard for their health or hard earned monies.

How do I make sense of my survey and observation? Well, there is a strong relationship between obesity and tendency to eat processed foods. And more importantly, obesity is correlated with lack of vegetable and fruit diets. Lesson: do not get lured with coupons and discounts of supermarkets and do your shopping in the periphery of the store rather than the interior of the store because it is better for your health.

Actually, we are very lucky in America because we have the nutritional and caloric contents labels. Let me show you how you could turn these labels into your advantage by reviewing with you the information on several products: some good, some bad, and some ugly. The following shopping examples never were a representation of my shopping habit for three main reasons:1) most of my foods consist of produce, grains, poultry, seafood, and meat; 2) this is not the scope of this book; 3) and finally, I want you to be an active learner by reading the labels in your own.

Let's start with Potato Chips.

1) **Frito-Lay's Classic Potato Chips:** 28 grams/serving (1 serving); 150 calories; 380 grams per package; total fat 39%, sat fat 14%, carbohydrates 13%, fiber 10%, sodium 2,400 mg, sugar 0 grams, and traces of vitamins and minerals. Ingredients: potatoes, sunflower oil, and salt.

2) **Doritos (Nacho Cheese):** 150 calories, 410 grams per package, total fat 12%, sat fat 7%, sodium 180 mg, carbohydrates 6%, fiber 6%, sugar 1 gram, protein 2 gram, and cholesterol 0 mg. Ingredients: vegetable oil, salt, cheddar cheese, **maltodextran**, wheat flour, MSG, butter milk, cottonseed oil, dextrose, yellow 6, yellow 5, and red 40.

If I were to choose between Frito-Lay's Classic Potato Chips and Doritos (Nacho Cheese) for my kids, I will choose Lay's, for the following reasons:

1) High sodium content (2,400 mg), high saturated fat (14%), and 380 grams /package for Frito-Lay's. Less ingredients, some trace elements and vitamins, and most of all no MSG, maltodextran, dextrose or vegetable oil.

2) **Matodextran,** MSG, butter milk, cottonseed oil, dextrose and inclusion of many food dyes such as yellow 6, yellow 5, and red 5 in Doritos (Nacho Cheese). I might say that Doritos tastes better!

Let's move to some snacks.

1) **Peanut Butter (Frito Lay's):** Sat fat 25%; calories 190; sodium 370 mg; sugar 3 grams; and some trace elements and vitamins.

2)**Natural Nut Harvest (Frito Lay's):** Calories 210; sat fat 12%; sodium 125 mg; fiber 5 grams; sugar 1 gram; and some trace elements and vitamins.

Peanut Butter (Frito Lay's) has high content of saturated fat (25%) and high sugar content (3 grams). Natural Nut Harvest is better because it has less sugar content and more fiber (5 grams).

Let's move to the chocolate section.

1)**Hershey's Milk Chocolate:** calories 400; calories from fat 210; sat fat 14 grams; trans fat 0 gram; cholesterol 15 mg; carbohydrates 42 grams; fiber 5 grams; and some iron and calcium. Ingredients: milk chocolate and vanilla.

2) **3 Musketeers:** Carbohydrates 400; Sat fat 4 grams; Cholesterol 5 mg; trans fat 0 grams; carbohydrates 35 grams; fiber 1 gram; and some trace elements and vitamins. Ingredients: hydrogenated palm kernel, milk chocolate, palm oil, cocoa powder and some flavors.

3)**Nestle® Babe Ruth:** Calories 250; sat fat 6 grams; trans fat 0 grams; cholesterol 0 mg; sodium 115 mg; fiber 1 gram; carbohydrates 33 grams; fiber 1 gram; and some trace elements of iron and calcium.

None of the chocolates above is my first choice because they do not have at least 60% of cocoa. If I have to choose between the three of them, I will choose Nestle® Babe Ruth because it has the least carbohydrate content per calories, and void of palm oil and cholesterol.

Finally, let's move to the Pringles section.

1) **Pringles- Light & fat-free**: fewer calories and made with olestra; calories 70; sodium 160 mg; carbohydrates 15 grams fiber 1 gram; and sugar 1 gram. Ingredients: In red background and hard to read, dries potato and olestra.

2)**Pringles Barbecue Flavored**: total fat 10 grams; sodium 160 mg; carbohydrates 14 grams; fiber 1 gram; sugar 1 gram; and some trace elements and vitamins. Ingredients: dried potato, cottonseed oil, paprika, MSG, and extract colors.

3)**Pringles- Sour Cream & Onion**: fat 10 grams (3 grams from saturated fat); sodium 180 mg; carbohydrates 14 grams; sugar 1 gram; and sodium 0 mg. Ingredients: dried potatoes, corn oil, cottonseed oil, MSG, partially hydrogenated and coconut oil.

If I have to choose between these three brands of Pringles, I would not choose Pringles with olestra because it sucks away all of the valuable fat-soluble vitamins, especially vitamin A. Moreover, olestra gives the stool the consistency of tea. The other two brands of Pringles are discarded because of their content of MSG; MSG, monosodium glutamate, is a flavor enhancer, and one of the food additives that I would rather not eat. If I were on weight-loss diet, I will pick Pringles-light &fat free and supplement the adverse effect of olestra by eating some carrots.

Many of the color additives in America require FDA certification and they come basically in two forms: Straight colors and lakes. Straight color additives are mostly water-soluble additives. Certain straight colors are used to make lake additives. Lake food additives are used in products in which bleaching or " bleeding" of color would pose problems, such as in cookie fillings, coated tablets, candies, chewing gums, and lipsticks. Here are some of the most common food and cosmetic additives used:

1) **Olestra**-although approved by FDA, it sucks away valuable nutrients and flushes them out of the body. Some of these nutrients are carotenoids that protect from cancer and ocular degeneration.

2) **Nitrite and Nitrate**- sodium nitrite and sodium nitrate are used to preserve meat. Nitrite reacts with secondary amines to form nitrosamines, extremely powerful cancer-causing chemicals such as stomach cancer.

3) **Monosodium Glutamate (MSG)** - is added to the flavor of protein-containing foods. Too much MSG can lead to headache, tightness in the chest and a burning sensation in the forearm.

4) **BHA and BHT**- these two closely related chemicals are added to oil-containing foods to retard rancidity (oxidation). The World Health Organization (WHO) considers BHA to be possibly carcinogenic to humans.

5) **Equal and NutraSweet**- Equal, Aspartame, a sugar substitute and should not be given to phenylketonurea (PKU) patients because some of them are born without the ability to metabolize phenylalanine; one of the two amino acids in aspartame.

6) **Sunnette or Sweet One**- is a sugar substitute found mostly in chewing gums, dry mixes of beverages, instant coffees and teas, gelatin deserts, puddings, and non-dairy creamers.

7)**Sulfites**- are used to keep cut fruits and vegetables looking fresh; prevent discoloration in apricots, raisins, and other dried fruits; control black spot in freshly caught shrimp; and prevent discoloration, bacterial growth, and fermentation in wine. US congress banned sulfites' use in 1985, but the ban does not cover fresh-cut potatoes, dried fruits and wines.

8) **FD& C Red No. 3**- although about one-third of its provisional uses is banned in 1990, FD&C Red No.3 is still permanently listed for use in foods and drugs, such as baked goods, cherries,

dairy products, dietary supplements, desserts, food seasonings, jams, and jellies.

9) **FD& C Yellow No.5**- this additive causes cancer in mammal studies, but causes allergic reactions in some people; FDA requires allergic reaction to be listed in food labels.

10) **Potassium Bromate**- is used to increase volume of bread and to produce bread with a fine crumb texture. Potassium bromate has been banned virtually worldwide except in Japan and the United States, but is rarely used in California because a cancer-warning is required on the label.

11) **de minimis non curat lex's dyes**- the maxim "de minimis non curat lex," means that the law does not concern itself with trifles. In short, FDA approved FD& C Orange Nos. 8 and 9 on this legal maxim. However, a year later, the US Court of Appeals for the District of Columbia ordered FDA to ban these additives.

12) **Maltodextran** (a sugar substitute) should be used in extremely small amounts.

I hope that you got a sense of the importance of reading food labels carefully. Let me summarize for you my recommendation about them:

a) Buy foods with ingredients you would use at home.

b) Avoid products with too many ingredients.

c) Watch out for saturated fats, partially hydrogenated fats, and trans- fats or oils.

d) Minimize consumption of products with MSG, BHA, BHT and aluminum because they pose health risk, in my opinion.

e) Check nutrition facts and adjust the arithmetic in some of them.

f) Use local, organic, produce if possible to avoid pesticides and other contaminants.

Chapter 11

Eating Out

"The art of printing secures us against the retro gradation of reason and information."

Thomas Jefferson

Despite the convenience of eating out, you cannot know how carefully these outlets choose their food; you can improve your chances of getting healthy food by making wise choices where to eat and what to order. I usually enjoy eating at restaurants because they usually offer heart-healthful main dishes. Luckily, we have a wide variety of cuisines to choose from; properly cooked- meat and vegetarian appetizers made with olive oil at Middle Eastern and Greek restaurants, stir-fried vegetables and seafood at Oriental ones, pasta with marinara sauce and fresh salad at Italian restaurants, and of course T-bone steaks and salad bars at American ones.

Usually the quality of most restaurants is often very good if they score 90 or better in the health department inspections. However, I do have some suggestions to get the best for your buck and belly.

a) Since portions of most restaurants are too large, consider splitting dishes with fellow dinners, take the excess home, or just leave it on the plate.

b) Choose brightly light over softly light dining areas.

c) Choose warmer dining areas over cold ones.

d) Choose conversation over music or TV to distract you from eating too much.

e) Avoid butter, cream-based soups, French fries, sauces, and high-glycemic breads.

f) Choose olive oil, vinegar or lemon over salad dressing.

g) Always have a fellow dinner to distract you from eating a lot or have a book or magazine to read.

h) Drink a 1/2 cup of water before eating.

i) Replace potato and rice with sautéed vegetables.

j)Order oil and vinegar at separate containers and pour it (them) yourself because relying on the wait staff or chef to do so gets you lots of unneeded calories (400 -500 extra) per side salad.

Items to Avoid in Restaurants

American: Fries and anything has Fries in name, mashed potatoes, and grilled cheese.

Middle Eastern/ Mediterranean: Phylo dough, meatballs, fried and breaded meals. Most Middle Eastern/Mediterranean food is healthy.

Italian: Fried calamari and zucchini, stuffed mushrooms, fettuccine Alfredo, baked ziti, anything with bread crumbs, and pizza with meat toppings and lots of cheese.

Mexican: Fried flour or corn made items such as tortilla, taco shells, sour cream, cheese, quesadillas, and lots of chalupas, nachos, ground beef or pork.

Oriental: Noodles because most are drenched in saturated fats; white rice; anything described as crispy or fried; Temperua; Tso's chicken, egg dishes, such as egg foo yong; and salty soups.

Luckily for me, studying and living in our nation's capital offers the finest cuisine in the world because those outlets compete to serve savvy diners and dignitaries from all over the world. As long as you are able to cough a hefty bill, you always find fine cuisines in Washington, D.C., especially at The George Washington University's Foggy Bottom campus, which is a walking distance from the White House and Capitol Hill.

When you have to eat out in fast food places, these are the best places for your heart with their caloric content in parenthesis. These items were chosen for their low cholesterol and sodium contents.

1) Main dishes

Arby's

Grilled Chicken deluxe (450)	BBQ vinaigrette (140)
Breast Fillet (540)	Italian, reduced cal (25)
Sub-Turkey (630)	Croutons -cheese/garlic (100)

Any combination of main dish and a salad dressing will give you around 600- 700 calories (that is more than a 1/3 of your daily allowance).

Burger King

BK Home-style Grilled (480)	Hamburger, double (450)
BK Veggie Burger w/out mayo (290)	Chicken Caesar (160)

Denny's

Chicken Grilled (520)	Turkey Multigrain (476)
Reuben (580)	the Super Bird (620)

Domino's Pizza

Thin Crust-Pizza with green pepper, mushroom, pineapple, olives, and onion

Dunk' Donuts

All bagels are okay (about 300).

Hardee's

Big Roast Beef (410)	Chicken Fillet (480)
Fisherman's Fillet (530)	Twist Cone (180)

Jack-in the-Box

Cheeseburger, double (410)   Hamburger w/cheese (390)

Chicken Sandwich (410)   Sourdough grilled chicken club (490)

KFC (the following sandwiches have about 60 mg cholesterol per each).

Original Recipe w/out sauce Sandwich (360)

Triple Crunch w/ out sauce (390)

Tender Roast w/ out sauce (270)

Triple Crunch Zinger w/out sauce (390)

McDonald's

Filet-O- Fish (470)   Quarter Pounder (430)

Chicken McGrill w/out mayo (300)   Chicken flatbread no sauce (460)

Subway (6") Deli Sandwiches

Veggie Delite (200)   Turkey Breast (254)

Roast Chicken Breast (311)   Subway Club (294)

Taco Bell

Chalupa nacho cheese: beef (380), Chicken (360), or steak (360)

Wendy's

Mandarin chicken with almond only (280) Chicken Breaded fillet (430)

Chicken Sandwich grilled (300)   Chicken Sandwich Spicy (430)

Whataburger

Chicken Sandwich grilled no / dressing (397)

Whataburger small bun, no oil (424)

Salad -grilled chicken (216)

2) Dressings (2 ounces)

Ranch (310), ranch-low fat (70), Thousand Island (160), French style-low fat (90), Oriental sesame (280), vinaigrette (220), vinaigrette-low fat (35), blue cheese (290), and Caesar (150).

3) Sides

Fries, Jr. (240), Fries regular (420), Fries large (560), Onion rings -large (464), onion rings regular (307), peppered gravy (3 ounces) 53, and Texas toast slice (137).

4) Condiments

American cheese (70), American cheese -Jr (45), Bacon -1 slice (20), honey mustard-1 1/2 tablespoon (5), pickles (0), and tomato- 1 slice (5).

Here are some words for the wise:

a) Be careful because some slight variations can make the difference between health and sickness.

b) Avoid side dishes, dressings, and condiments because they are all loaded with fats and simple sugars, and they are often loaded with calories more than the main dishes.

c) Choose low-calorie dressing, not low-fat because low -fat dressings are loaded with HFCS (fructose), which has plenty of calories and tricks your body into staying hungry.

d) Sorry, I could not find any healthy breakfast menus in any fast food place. But simple Bacon, cheese, egg sandwich will do- whether at home or at fast food outlets.

Chapter 12

Food-borne Diseases

"Agony Purifies the Human Soul."

Dad

Food-borne disease is caused by consuming contaminated foods or beverages with pathogens or poisonous chemicals. More than 250 different food-borne diseases are caused by bacteria, viruses, and parasites that can be food-borne. Other borne-diseases result from harmful poisons as poisonous mushrooms. These different diseases have many different symptoms by a microbe or a toxin that enters the body through the gastrointestinal tract, and often causes nausea, vomiting, abdominal cramps and diarrhea as common symptoms in many food-borne diseases. Many microbes can spread in more than one way; for example *Escherichia coli* infections can spread through contaminated food, contaminated drinking water, contaminated swimming water, and between toddlers at a day care center. Therefore, the measures to combat food-borne diseases range from removing contaminated food from stores, chlorinating a swimming pool, or closing a child day care center.

Campylobacter, *Salmonella*, and *E. coli* bacteria and a group of viruses called calicivirus, also known as the <u>Norwalk</u> and Norwalk-like viruses are the most common causes of food-borne diseases. *Campylobacter* is a bacterial pathogen that causes fever, diarrhea, and abdominal cramps, and it's the most commonly identified bacterial cause of diarrheal illness in the world. These bacteria live in the intestines of healthy birds, and most raw poultry meat has *Campylobacter* on it. Eating undercooked chicken or other food that has been contaminated with juices dripping from raw chicken is the most frequent source of this infection. _Salmonella_ is also a bacterium that is widespread in the intestines of birds, reptiles and mammals. It can spread to humans via a variety of different foods of animal origin. The illness it causes, salmonellosis, typically includes fever, diarrhea and abdominal cramps. _E. coli_ causes human illness after consumption of food or water that has been contaminated with microscopic amounts of cow feces. The illness is often a severe and bloody diarrhea and painful abdominal cramps, without much fever. In 3% to 5% of cases, a complication called hemolytic uremic syndrome (HUS) can occur several weeks after the initial symptoms. These severe complications include temporary anemia, profuse bleeding, and kidney failure.

Calicivirus, or Norwalk-like virus is an extremely common cause of food-borne illness; it causes an acute gastrointestinal illness, usually with more vomiting than diarrhea that resolves within two days. Unlike many food-borne pathogens that have animal reservoirs, it's believed that Norwalk-like viruses spread primarily from one infected person to another. Some common diseases are occasionally food-borne although they are usually transmitted by other routes. These include infections caused by _Shigella_, _hepatitis A_, and the parasites _Giardia lamblia_ and _Cryptosporidia_. Even strep throats have been transmitted occasionally through food.

Some food-borne diseases are caused by the presence of a toxin in the food that was produced by a microbe in the food. For example, the bacterium *Staphylococcus aureus* can grow in some foods and produce a toxin that causes intense vomiting. The rare but deadly disease botulism occurs when the bacterium <u>*Clostridium botulinum*</u> grows and produces a powerful paralytic toxin in foods. These toxins can produce illness even if the microbes that produced them are no longer there. Other toxins and poisonous chemicals cause food-borne illness; for example, from a pesticide inadvertently added to a food, or a naturally poisonous substances used to prepare a meal. Many people become ill after mistaking poisonous mushrooms for safe species, or after eating poisonous reef fishes.

Many food-borne microbes are present in healthy animals (usually in their intestines) raised for food. Meat and poultry carcasses can become contaminated during slaughter by contact with small amounts of intestinal contents. Similarly, fresh fruits and vegetables can be contaminated if they are washed or irrigated with water that is contaminated with animal manure or human sewage. Some types of <u>*Salmonella*</u> can infect a hen's ovary so that the internal contents of a normal looking egg can be contaminated with <u>*Salmonella*</u> even before the shell in formed. Oysters and other filter feeding shellfish can concentrate <u>*Vibrio*</u> bacteria that are naturally present in sea water, or other microbes that are present in human sewage dumped into the sea. The good news is most microbes are killed by heat; an internal temperature above 160°F, or 78°C, for even a few seconds is sufficient to kill parasites, viruses or bacteria, except for the <u>*Clostridium*</u> bacteria, which produce a heat-resistant form called a spore.

Clostridium spores are killed only at a temperature above boiling (212ºF or 100ºC.). This is why canned foods must be cooked to a high temperature under pressure as part of the canning process. However, toxins produced by bacteria vary in their sensitivity to heat. The staphylococcal toxin which causes vomiting is not inactivated even if it is boiled. Fortunately, the potent toxin that causes botulism is completely inactivated by boiling. Raw meat, raw eggs, unpasteurized milk, and raw shellfish are the most common sources of food-borne diseases; further, food-borne disease are transmitted through food processing or through preparation from kitchen ware or people. Consumption of raw fruits and vegetables is of a particular concern because washing only decreases but does not eliminate contamination. Outbreaks have been traced to fresh fruits and vegetables that were processed under less than sanitary conditions because the quality of the water used for washing and chilling the produce after it's harvested. Fresh manure fertilization and pasteurization of fruit juices or milk and sprouting conditions as in alfalfa sprouts and other raw sprouts pose a particular challenge because they are eaten without further cooking because a few bacteria present on the seeds can grow to high numbers of pathogens on the sprouts.

CDC estimates that each year roughly 1 out of 6 Americans gets sick; the great majority of these cases is mild and causes symptoms for only a day or two. The most severe cases tend to occur in the very old, the very young, those who have an illness already that reduces their immune system function, and in healthy people exposed to a very high dose of an organism. Food--borne illness' outbreak occurs when a group of people consume the same contaminated food and two or more of people come down with the same illness. For an outbreak to occur, something must contaminate a batch of food that is eaten by a group of people. A contaminated food may be left out at a room temperature for many hours, allowing the bacteria to multiply to high numbers, and then be insufficiently cooked to kill the bacteria.

Common -sense precautions to reduce the risk of food-borne diseases:

<u>**COOK**</u> meat, poultry and eggs thoroughly and use a thermometer to measure the internal temperature of meat to assure that it's cooked sufficiently to kill bacteria. For example, ground beef should be cooked to an internal temperature of 160º F and eggs should be cooked until the yolk is firm.

<u>**SEPARATE**</u>: Do not cross-contaminate one food with another; wash hands, utensils, and cutting boards after they have been in contact with raw meat or poultry and before they touch another food.

<u>**CHILL**</u>: Refrigerate leftovers promptly. Bacteria can grow quickly at room temperature, so refrigerate leftover foods if they are not going to be eaten within 4 hours.

<u>**CLEAN**</u>: Wash produce and rinse fresh fruits and vegetables in running tap water to remove visible dirt and grime. Remove and discard the outermost leaves of a head of lettuce or cabbage.

<u>**REPORT**</u>: Report suspected food-borne illnesses to health departments and produce stores to prevent subsequent sales and sickness of others.

Some persons at particularly high risk should take more precautions.

- Pregnant women, the elderly, and those weakened immune systems are at higher risk for severe infections such as _Listeria_ and should be particularly careful not to consume undercooked animal products.

- A bottle-fed infant is at higher risk for severe infections with _Salmonella_ or other bacteria that can grow in a bottle of warm formula if it's left at room temperature for many hours

- Persons with liver disease are susceptible to infections with a rare but dangerous microbe called _Vibrio vulnificus_, found in oysters.

Other **common** bacterial food-borne pathogens:

- _Bacillus cereus_, _Escherichia coli_, other virulence properties, such as enteroinvasive (EIEC), enteropathogenic (EPEC), enterotoxigenic (ETEC), enteroaggregative (EAEC or EAgEC)

- _Listeria monocytogenes_, _Shigella_ spp., _Staphylococcus aureus_, _Staphylococcal enteritis_, _Streptococcus_, _Vibrio cholerae_, including O1 and non-O1, _Vibrio parahaemolyticus_, _Vibrio vulnificus_, _Yersinia enterocolitica_ and _Yersinia pseudotuberculosis_

Less common bacterial agents:_Brucella_ spp., _Corynebacterium ulcerans_, _Coxiella burnetii_ or Q fever, _Plesiomonas shigelloides_

Mycotoxins and alimentary mycotoxicoses

The term **alimentary mycotoxicoses** refers to the effect of poisoning by Mycotoxins through food consumption. Mycotoxins sometimes have important effects on human and animal health. For example, an outbreak which occurred in the UK in 1960 caused the death of 100,000 turkeys, which had consumed aflatoxin-contaminated peanut meal. In Russia during World War II, 5000 people died due to Alimentary Toxic Aleukia (ALA). The common food-borne Mycotoxins are listed below:

- Aflatoxins – originated from Aspergillus parasiticus and Aspergillus flavus. They are frequently found in tree nuts, peanuts, maize, sorghum and other oilseeds, including corn and cottonseeds. The pronounced forms of aflatoxins are those of B1, B2, G1, and G2, amongst which aflatoxin B1 predominantly targets the liver, which will result in necrosis, cirrhosis, and carcinoma.[10][11] In the US, the acceptable level of total aflatoxins in foods is less than 20 µg/kg, except for aflatoxin M1 in milk, which should be less than 0.5 µg/kg. The official document can be found at FDA's website.

- Altertoxins – are those of Alternariol (AOH), Alternariol methyl ether (AME), Altenuene (ALT), Altertoxin-1 (ATX-1), Tenuazonic acid (TeA) and Radicinin (RAD), originated from Alternaria spp. Some of the toxins can be present in sorghum, ragi, wheat and tomatoes. Some research has shown that the toxins can be easily cross-contaminated between grain commodities, suggesting that manufacturing and storage of grain commodities is a critical practice to combat food-borne illnesses.

- Citrinin, Citreoviridin, Cyclopiazonic acid, Cytochalasins, Ergot alkaloids / Ergopeptine alkaloids – Ergotamine

- Fumonisins – Crop corn can be easily contaminated by the fungi Fusarium moniliforme, and its Fumonisin B1 will cause Leukoencephalomalacia (LEM) in horses, pulmonary edema syndrome (PES) in pigs, liver cancer in rats and Esophageal cancer in humans. For human and animal health, both the FDA and the EC have regulated the content levels of toxins in food and animal feed.

- Fusaric acid, Fusarochromanone , Kojic acid, Lolitrem alkaloids Moniliformin, 3-Nitropropionic acid, Nivalenol

- Ochratoxins – In Australia, The Limit Of Reporting (LOR) level for Ochratoxin A (OTA) analyses in 20th Australian Total Diet Survey was 1 µg/kg, whereas the EC restricts the content of OTA to 5 µg/kg in cereal commodities, 3 µg/kg in processed products, and 10 µg/kg in dried vine fruits.

- Patulin – Currently, this toxin has been advisably regulated on fruit products. The EC and the FDA have limited patulin levels to 50 µg/kg or less for fruit juice and fruit nectar, while limits of 25 µg/kg for solid-contained fruit products, and 10 µg/kg for baby foods were specified by the EC.

- Phomopsins, Sporidesmin A, Sterigmatocystin, Tremorgenic mycotoxins – Five of them have been reported to be associated with molds found in fermented meats. These are Fumitremorgen B, Paxilline, Penitrem A, Verrucosidin, and Verruculogen.

- Trichothecenes – sourced from Cephalosporium, Fusarium, Myrothecium, Stachybotrys and Trichoderma. The toxins are usually found in molded maize, wheat, corn, peanuts and rice, or animal feed of hay and straw. Four trichothecenes, T-2 toxin, HT-2 toxin, diacetoxyscirpenol (DAS) and deoxynivalenol (DON) have been most commonly encountered by humans and animals. The consequences of oral intake of, or dermal exposure to, the toxins will result in alimentary toxic aleukia, neutropenia, aplastic anemia, thrombocytopenia and/or skin irritation. In 1993, the FDA issued a document for the content limits of DON in food and animal feed at an advisory level. In 2003, US published a patent that is very promising for farmers to produce a trichothecene-resistant crop.

Parasites

Most food-borne parasites are zoonoses.

- Platyhelminthes: *Diphyllobothrium* sp., *Nanophyetus* sp., *Taenia saginata*, *Taenia solium*, *Fasciola hepatica*, *Tapeworm and Flatworm*

  - Nematode: *Anisakis* sp., *Ascaris lumbricoides*, *Eustrongylides* sp., *Trichinella spiralis*, *Trichuris trichiura*

  - Protozoa:

    o *Acanthamoeba* and other free-living amoebae, *Cryptosporidium parvum*, *Cyclospora cayetanensis*, *Entamoeba histolytica*, *Giardia lamblia* , *Giardia lamblia*,

93

Sarcocystis hominis, Sarcocystis suihominis, _Toxoplasma_
gondii

Natural toxins

Several foods can naturally contain toxins, many of which are not produced by bacteria. Plants in particular may be toxic, but naturally poisonous animals are rare. Examples of plant toxins are capsaicin in chili peppers and pungent sulfur compounds in garlic and onions. Most animal poisons are not synthesized by the animal, but acquired by eating poisonous plants to which the animal is immune or by a bacterial action.

- Alkaloids, Ciguatera poisoning, Grayanotoxin (honey intoxication), Mushroom toxins, Phytohaemagglutinin (red kidney bean poisoning; destroyed by boiling), Pyrrolizidine alkaloids

- Shellfish toxin, including paralytic shellfish poisoning, diarrheic shellfish poisoning, neurotoxin shellfish poisoning, amnesic shellfish poisoning and ciguatera fish poisoning, Scombrotoxin, Tetrodotoxin (fugu fish poisoning)

Some plants contain substances which are toxic in large doses but have therapeutic properties in appropriate dosages, such as:

- Foxglove contains cardiac glycosides.

- Poisonous hemlock (conium) has medicinal uses.

Chapter 13

The Twelve-Week Program

"People react to fear, not love. They don't teach that in Sunday school, but it is true."

Richard Nixon

In this program you will find three steps to weight loss:

1. Find your desirable BMI (weight),

2. Determine your caloric needs for weight loss, and

3. Follow the diet plan to achieve your desired weight.

Step One: Find your BMI (weight)

Height	Weight (pounds)													
BMI	19	20	21	22	23	24	25	26	27	28	29	30	35	40
4' 10"	91	96	100	105	110	115	120	124	130	134	139	144	160	192
4' 11'	94	99	104	109	114	119	124	128	133	138	143	148	173	198
5' 0"	97	102	107	112	118	123	128	133	138	143	148	153	179	204
5' 1"	100	106	111	116	122	127	132	137	143	148	153	159	185	211
5' 2"	104	109	115	120	126	131	136	142	147	153	158	164	191	218
5' 3"	107	113	118	124	130	135	141	146	152	158	163	169	197	225
5' 4"	110	116	122	128	_134_	140	145	151	157	163	169	174	204	232
5' 5"	114	120	126	132	~~138~~	145	150	156	162	168	174	180	210	240
5' 6"	118	124	130	136	_142_	148	155	161	167	173	179	186	216	247
5' 7"	121	128	135	141	147	153	159	166	172	178	185	191	223	255
5' 8"	125	131	138	145	151	158	165	171	177	184	190	197	230	262
5' 9"	128	136	142	149	155	162	169	176	182	189	196	203	236	270
5' 10"	132	139	146	153	160	_167_	174	181	188	195	202	207	243	278
5' 11"	136	143	150	157	_165_	_172_	179	186	193	200	208	215	250	286
6' 0"	140	147	154	162	_169_	177	184	191	199	206	213	221	258	294
6' 1"	144	151	159	166	174	182	189	197	201	212	219	228	265	302
6' 2"	148	156	163	171	179	186	194	202	210	218	225	233	272	311
6' 3"	152	160	167	176	184	192	200	208	216	224	232	240	279	319
6' 4"	156	164	172	185	189	197	205	213	221	230	238	246	287	328
6' 5'	160	169	177	185	194	202	211	219	228	236	244	253	295	337

Note: underlined BMI represents males and strikethrough BMI represents females of the Ibrahim family. (Kilogram=2.2 pounds.)

What is your family BMI? Write it down; it is part of the psychological face-off of your overweight or obesity problem.

Step Two: What is your goal?

Set a realistic goal for weight loss to avoid disappointment. For example, if you have not weighed less than 175 pounds since you were 16, a goal of 140 pounds may be unrealistic. Instead of setting a goal that you cannot reach, choose a more achievable goal, such as a 160- pound goal. For example, a 210-pound, for 5' 10" man would still be considered overweight; at 190 pounds (a 10 % weight loss), he would have a substantially lower risk for health problems. Just weigh yourself daily, at the same time, wearing the same amount of clothing.

Do not track your weight daily but weekly to avoid day-to-day fluctuations.

Step Three: What is your metabolic base for weight loss?

1) If you have a healthy BMI, you are eating the right amount for your weight. If you are overweight (BMI= 25- 29.9), subtract 400 calories from your daily allowances. If you are obese (BMI =30 or above), subtract 600 calories from your daily allowances.

2) Be sure to adjust for starting a physical activity program in your life. Use the values given before as a guide to approximate your physical activity's caloric needs.

3) You can estimate your Resting Metabolic Rate (RMR) by multiplying your desired weight in pounds by 8 and add 200. Although this method is variable, it is the best in hand.

4) To estimate your calories from physical activity, look up the values given before or a comparable value close to your physical activity.

5) If you want to weigh 200 pounds and do walking for 2 miles daily, your basic calories used are 8 x 200= 1,600 +200= 1,800.

1,800 + 200 calories (for walking 2 miles) = 2,000.

So to maintain your desired weight, you would need about 2,000 calories a day. To lose a pound a week, you would need to decrease your caloric intake by 400 calories a day (if overweight), and by 600 calories a day (if obese). Do not worry because your body will make up the difference between your caloric intake and your caloric needs from your omentum (fat storage). Actually, your omentum evolved genetically to serve you with needed calories by burning the stored fat. It is like a safeguard against starvation or lack of food because of harsh weather conditions in earlier times of human evolution. 20,000 years ago, when our ancestors chased other animals and nuts for food when food resources were scarce and life was tough because of fierce competition, lack of advanced tools, and harsh weather conditions.

The other way to do that is to increase your physical activity by 400 calories a day (if overweight) and by 600 calories a day (if obese), or a combination of the two, food and physical activity.

6) When you lose weight, you daily caloric intake will decrease accordingly. Do the caloric adjustments at the end of the week after weighing yourself and calculation of desired weight.

7) Do not use the waist size method as a guide because it is not accurate; especially for the pear-shaped bodies (obese hips and butts).

The Two- Week Meal Program

All these menus or recipes are designed for 1,700 calories a day per person, but you can decrease or increase your physical activity to make up for the lost or extra calories that fit your desired body weight.

Saturday

1. **Walk** for 2 miles (about 30 minutes). Only actual walking time counts.

2. **Stretch** for 5 minutes after walking to keep your muscles flexible and help you refocus and cope with cravings.

3. **Clean** your fridge of saturated, *trans* fats, processed and simple foods, and enriched flours. Do not give these nutritional felons to charity; just dump them in the garbage.

4. **Go shopping** with a previously written food list and read the label of everything you buy. It is time consuming at the first time, but you will eventually learn to buy the healthy items only. Buy your shopping needs for a week.

Day 1: Sunday

Breakfast:

> **Cereal:** Kashi Go Lean Crunch (1 cup- 190 Cal)+ 1 cup of 2% A&D fortified milk (137 Cal)+ 1 fistful of your favorite fruit (about 70-80 Cal) or a 1/2 dozen nuts (180 Cal). Take 1 cup of green tea, decaffeinated coffee without sugar or just plain water. Breakfast Calories= 400- 500.

Lunch:

> **Salmon Salad**: 1/2 dozen chopped nuts (180 Cal)+ 1 cup of chopped vegetables of your choice (80 Cal)+4.5 ounces of Bumble Bee canned salmon (180 Cal)+ 1/2 teaspoon of olive oil - dressing (60 Cal)+ 1 fistful of your favorite fruit (70- 80 Cal).

> Take 1 cup of green tea, decaffeinated coffee without sugar, or two cups of plain water. Lunch Calories: 580.

Dinner:

> **Chicken:** 4 ounces of breast chicken grilled or baked and rubbed lightly with olive oil and cooked with sliced red onion, mushroom, and celery (350 cal) + 1 medium sweet potato (grilled or baked) brushed lightly with olive oil (150 cal) + 1/2 cup cooked baby lima beans (50 cal).

> Take 1 cup of green tea and plenty of water. Dinner calories: 550.

Day 2: Monday

Breakfast:

Omelet: 2 egg whites and a whole egg (scrambled) in canola oil   (280 Cal) + 1 slices of Oat bran (85 Cal) + 1 fistful of your favorite fruit (about 70-80 Cals) or a 1/2 dozen of your favorite   nuts (180 Cals).

Take 1 cup of green tea, decaffeinated coffee without sugar or just plain water.

Breakfast calories: 600.

Lunch:

Tuna: fish 2 ounces or 1/4 cup-canned in spring water or oil-   drained (110 Cal)+ 2 chopped hard-boiled egg whites (130 Cal)   tossed with 1 teaspoon of olive oil (120 Cal) for dressing on a bed   of lettuce + 1 fistful of your favorite fruit (70- 80 cal)+ 1 slice of   low- cottage cheese (70 cal).

Take 1 cup of green tea, decaffeinated coffee without sugar, or just plain water.

Lunch calories: 500.

Dinner:

Veal: 1 cup of Shiitake mushroom sautéed in olive oil and garlic or red onion (140 cal) with 4 ounces of grilled lean veal chop   rubbed   lightly with olive oil (240) +1/2 cup of cooked frozen   green peas (100 cal).

Dessert: 1/2 serving (equivalent to the size of a half medium   apple) Cheesecake-raspberry   crumble (Mountain House)   (75   cal).

Take 1 cup of green tea and plenty of water.

Dinner calories: 550.

Day 3: Tuesday

Breakfast:

Soy Spread (soy Wonder): 2 tablespoons on 2 slices of 100% whole-wheat or oat bran bread (170 Cal) of bread + 170 Cal of Soy spread) + 1 fistful of your favorite fruit (70-80 Cal).

Take 1 cup of green tea, decaffeinated coffee without sugar, or just plain water.

Breakfast Calories= 420- 450.

Lunch:

Hamburger: 2 pieces of grilled hamburgers -White Castle (270 Cal) on whole-grain bun (155 Cal) with one melted cheese (70 cal), and 2 slices of tomatoes (20 Cal) and celery sticks.

Take 1 cup of green tea, decaffeinated coffee without sugar, or just plain water. Take

Lunch calories: 510.

Dinner:

Lamb: 4 ounces of lamb chops or lamb sirloin steak grilled with eggplant slices and brushed lightly with olive oil (300 cal)+ 2 cups of steamed fresh broccoli (50 cal)+ 1 cup of mixed salad greens with tomato chunks and marinated artichoke hearts and tossed with olive oil and vinegar (120 cal).

Dessert: Yogurt-Yoplait Light -6 ounces- (100 cal).

Take 1 cup of green tea and plenty of water.

Dinner calories: 570.

Day 4: Wednesday

Breakfast:

Bagel: Wild berry blueberry 1 piece (340 Cal) or Cinnamon raisin -Crusty (260) + 1 fistful of your favorite fruit (70- 80 Cal).1 cup of green tea, decaffeinated coffee without sugar, or just plain water. You may add a 1 cup of 2% A& D fortified milk to add 137 calories for total calories of 480

Breakfast Calories= 480.

Lunch:

Roast Beef: 4 slices of Healthy Choice Whole Muscle ,0.75 ounce each, (100 cal) on 2 slices of 100% whole-grain or oat bran toasted bread (170 cal) with mustard, lettuce, dill pickles, and olives (80 cal).

Take 1 fistful of your favorite fruit of the season (70-80 cal).

Take 1 cup of green tea, decaffeinated coffee without sugar, or   just plain water.

Loch calories: 420.

Dinner:

Fish: a package of Freezer Queen Meal fish sticks, 6.5 ounces, steamed or microwave with 2 cups of yellow pepper, red onion, broccoli florets, and garlic (450 cal)+ 1 cup of fresh spinach salad tossed with olive oil, red wine, vinegar, and mustard (100 cal).

Take 1 cup of green tea and plenty of water.

Dinner calories: 550.

Day 5: Thursday

Breakfast:

Eggroll: Yu Sing (chicken) 2 egg rolls (360 Cal) +1 cup of orange juice with pulp (110 Cal).

Take 1 cup of green tea, decaffeinated coffee without sugar, or just plain water.

Breakfast calories= 460.

Lunch:

Turkey bologna: 3 slices of Louis Rich (1 ounce each) (150 Cal) and 2 slices of Swiss cheese (140 cal) on whole-grain bun (155 cal) with mustard, lettuce, and 1 slice of tomato (30 Cal). 1 fistful of your favorite fruit equals (70- 80 Cal).

Take 1 cup of green tea, decaffeinated coffee without sugar, or just plain water.

Lunch calories: 550.

Dinner:

Ground Beef:4 ounces of lean ground beef (300 cal) cooked in   Contadina's tomato sauce-no sugar added+ Whole-green pasta   sprinkled   with   Romano   or Parmesan cheese (200 cal)+ 2 cups of   salad   greens with snow peas, roasted pine nuts, and a dressing of   olive oil, balsamic vinegar, and a dash of mustard(100 cal).

Take 1 cup of green tea and plenty of water.

Dinner calories: 600.

Day 6: Friday

Breakfast:

> **Turkey:** 3 slices of turkey bologna (160 Cal) + 2 slices of 100% whole- wheat or oat bran bread (170 Cal) + a 1/2 dozen of nuts (180 cal).

> Take 1 cup of green tea, decaffeinated coffee without sugar, or just plain water.

> Breakfast calories= 500.

Lunch:

> **Chicken:** 2 pieces of grilled chicken breast patty-Banquet (210   cal) on whole-wheat bun (155 cal) with lettuce, tomatoes,   mustard, and olives (80 cal) + 1 cup of orange or grapefruit (130   cal).

> Take 1 cup of green tea, decaffeinated coffee without sugar, or   just plain water.

> Lunch calories: 560.

Dinner:

> **Pork Chops:** 4 ounces of pork chops sautéed with sliced onions in 2 teaspoons of olive oil (300 cal) + Red kidney beans cooked with chopped onions, and garlic in olive or canola oil (100 cal) + 1/4 cup of brown rice cooked with chicken broth (150 cal) + 1 cup of artichoke, served with a dip of olive oil, garlic salt, and lemon   juice   (100 cal).

> Take 1 cup of green tea and plenty of water.

> Dinner calories: 650.

Day 7: Saturday

Breakfast:

Oatmeal: 1 cup of oatmeal (140 Cal) with 1 cup of 2% A& D fortified milk (137 Cal) + 1 cup of grapefruit (Tropicana calcium) or orange juice (130 Cal).

Take 1 cup of green tea, decaffeinated coffee without sugar, or just plain water.

Breakfast calories= 400.

Lunch:

Ham: 4 Slices of Healthy Choice Virginia ham (120 Cal) or 3 slices of Deli fat-free ham (150 cal) +2 slices of Swiss -Kraft singles (140 Cal) on whole-wheat bun (155 cal) with mustard, lettuce, red onion, and 2 slices of tomatoes (130 cal).

Take 1 cup of green tea, decaffeinated coffee without sugar, or just plain water.

Lunch calories: 550.

Dinner:

Venison: 4 ounces of venison sautéed in 1 cup of shiitake mushroom, red onion, and yellow pepper (300 cal)+ 1 cup of fresh cauliflower steamed with tomato and dressed with melted blue cheese (150 cal) + 1 cup of split pea as a soup in chicken broth with black pepper (100 cal).

Dessert: 1/4 cup of Yogurt Ice cream with no added sugar (50 cal).

Take 1 cup of green tea and plenty of water.

Dinner calories: 600.

Day 8: Sunday

Breakfast:

> **Pancakes:** 1/2 cup of Arrowhead Mills buckwheat pancakes (280 Cal) + 1/4 cup of Smucker's blueberry syrup (210 cal).
>
> Take 1 cup of green tea, decaffeinated coffee without sugar, or just plain water.
>
> Breakfast calories= 500.

Lunch:

> **Nut Salad:**1/2 dozen of chopped nuts (180 cal) +1 cup of salad greens (70 cal)+ 2 patties of grilled breast chicken - Banquet(220 cal) + yogurt-Dannon La Creme-4 ounces (140 cal).
>
> Take 1 cup of green tea, decaffeinated coffee without sugar, or just plain water.
>
> Lunch calories: 600.

Dinner:

> **Hawaiian:** 1/2 pie (6") of Contessa pizza with ham and shrimp   (450 cal) +1 cup of grapefruit or orange juice with pulp or 2%   A& D fortified milk (130 cal).
>
> Take 1 cup of green tea and plenty of   water.
>
> Dinner calories: 580.

Day 9: Monday

Breakfast:

>**Fruit Salad:** 1 medium banana sliced (105 Cal) + 1 cup of blueberry (90 cal) + 1/2 dozen nuts (180 cal).
>
>Take 1 cup of green tea, decaffeinated coffee without sugar, or just plain water.
>
>Breakfast calories= 400.

Lunch:

>**Peanut Butter:**2 tablespoons of Chunky /Crunchy Peter Pan peanut butter (190 cal) on whole-wheat bun or 1 slice of 100% whole-wheat or oat bran toasted bread (170 Cal)+ 1 fistful of your favorite fruit (70-80 cal) +1/2 dozen chopped nuts (180 cal). Take 1 cup of green tea, decaffeinated coffee without sugar, or just plain water.
>
>Lunch calories: 600.

Dinner:

>**Shrimp:** 4 ounces of raw shrimp grilled with lemon (120 cal) + 2 cups of steamed broccoli and yellow squash (70 cal) + 1/2 cup of whole-wheat pasta with tomato sauce and basil sautéed in olive oil and sprinkled with Romano or Parmesan cheese (210) + 1 cup of mixed salad greens with olive oil, red wine, and a dash of mustard (100 cal).
>
>**Dessert:** 1/4 cup of Sugar-free ice cream (75 cal).
>
>Take 1 cup of green tea and plenty of water.
>
>Dinner calories: 575.

Day 10: Tuesday

Breakfast:

> **Crackers:** graham cracker 8 pieces (130 cal) + 1 cup of 2% A&D fortified milk (137 Cal) + 1cup of grapefruit (Tropicana calcium) or orange juice (130 cal).
>
> Take 1 cup of green tea, decaffeinated coffee without sugar, or just plain water.
>
> Breakfast calories= 400.

Lunch:

> **Pizza:**1/2 pie of artichoke heart-Wolfgang Puck's pizza (340 cal)+ 1 cup of grapefruit (130 cal)+ 1 yogurt Dannon La Creme-4 ounces (140 Cal).
>
> Take 1 cup of green tea, decaffeinated coffee without sugar, or just plain water.
>
> Lunch calories: 610.

Dinner:

> **Steak:** 4 ounces of New York strip or lean sirloin steak rubbed lightly with olive oil and grilled (400 cal) + 1 cup of fresh mushroom (shiitake) sautéed in 1/2 teaspoon of olive oil with garlic and red onion (60 cal) + 1 cup of spinach with 2 slices of ripe tomato with 1 slice of mozzarella cheese with dressing of olive oil, vinegar, and a dash of mustard (150 cal).
>
> Take 1 cup of green tea and plenty of water.
>
> Dinner calories: 610.

Day 11: Wednesday

Breakfast:

Walnut Spread: Walnut butter-2 tablespoons (170 Cal) on 2   slices of 100% whole-wheat or oat bran toasted bread (170 Cal) + 1 fistful of your favorite fruit (70- 80 Cal).

Take 1 cup of green tea, decaffeinated coffee without sugar, or just plain water.

Breakfast calories= 410.

Lunch:

Chicken Nuggets: 7 ounces of Morton nuggets (340 cal) + 1 cup of salad (80 cal) + 1 yogurt Dannon La Creme-4 ounces (140   Cal) + 1 fistful of your favorite fruit (70- 80 Cal).

Take 1 cup of green tea, decaffeinated coffee without sugar, or just plain water.

Lunch calories: 550.

Dinner:

Fajita: one jalapeno steak- Hot Pockets (330 cal) + 1 cup of   grapefruit or orange juice with pulp or 2% A& D fortified milk (130 cal).

Dessert: 1/2 cup of Sugar-free ice cream (150 cal).

Take 1 cup of green tea and plenty of water.

Dinner calories: 580.

Day 12: Thursday

Breakfast:

Soy milk: Kellog's Mueslix -2/3 cup (200 cal)+ 1 cup of 2% A &D fortified milk (137 cal)+ 2 tablespoons of Soy beverage –Soy Nilla (50 Cal).

Take 1 cup of green tea, decaffeinated coffee without sugar, or just plain water.

Breakfast calories: 420.

Lunch:

Fish Fillet: 2 pieces of Gorton's fish fillets (270 cal) on whole- wheat bun (155 cal) with tomatoes, mustard, lettuce and olives (100 cal).

Take 1 cup of green tea, decaffeinated coffee without sugar, or just plain water.

Lunch calories: 530.

Dinner:

Gyros: combine 2 ounces of plain yogurt, 1/2 cup chopped seeded cucumber, 1/2 teaspoon finely chopped onion, and minced garlic clove, 1/4 pound of ground beef, with oregano, salt, and pepper in a bowl and mix well. Cover and refrigerate for 20 minutes, take it out and shape into a patty. Grill covered, over medium-hot heat for 10-12 minutes, or until no longer pink- turning once. Stuff into 1 pita bread; add lettuce, tomato and onion (450 cal).

Dessert: 1/2 cup of yogurt (sugar-free) (130 cal).

Take 1 cup of green tea and plenty of water.

Dinner calories: 580.

Day 13: Friday

Breakfast:

Croissant: 1 piece of Croissant -French style (170 Cal) +2 egg   whites and a whole egg (180 Cal) cooked in canola oil+ 1 fistful   of your favorite fruits (70-80 Cal) or 1 cup of grapefruit (130   Cal).

Take 1 cup of green tea, decaffeinated coffee without sugar, or   just plain water.

Breakfast calories= 480.

Lunch:

Falafel: Casbah, 1.5 ounces package of falafel mix makes 5 patties fried in canola oil (230 cal) with 1 cup of salad greens and olives(120 cal) and 1 cup of grapefruit or orange juice w/pulp   (130 cal).

Take 1 cup of green tea, decaffeinated coffee without sugar, or just plain water. Lunch calories: 480.

Dinner:

Lasagna: In a saucepan combine 1/4 cup of beef sauce, 1/2 can of tomato pasta and 1/2 teaspoon of basil and brings to a boil; reduce heat. Cover and simmer for 5 minutes. Combine 1/4 cup of small-curd cottage cheese and 3 egg-whites and mix well. Spoon   some   of   the meat sauce into a greased baking dish, layer with 3   boiled noodles, half of the cottage cheese mixture and 1/4 cup   mozzarella cheese. Repeat layers; top with remaining meat sauce and mozzarella. Cover and bake at 350⁰ for 20-25 minutes. Uncover; sprinkle with Parmesan cheese and bake for 10-12   minutes or until blobby and the cheese melted. Let stand for 10 minutes   before eating.

Dessert: 1/2 cup of grapefruit (65 cal).

Take 1 cup of green tea and plenty of water.

Dinner calories: 600.

Day 14: Saturday

Breakfast:

Fish: 2 pieces of Gorton's Grilled fillets (220 Cal) + 2 slices of   100% whole-wheat or oat bran bread (170 cal) + 1 fistful of your favorite fruits (70- 80 Cal).

Take 1 cup of green tea, decaffeinated coffee without sugar, or just plain water.

Breakfast calories: 440.

Lunch:

Veggie Burger: 2 patties of veggie burger -Dr.Praeger's (200 cal) on whole-wheat bun (155 cal) with mustard, lettuce, 1 slice of tomatoes, and olives (100 cal) + 1 fistful of your favorite fruit (70-80 cal).

Take 1 cup of green tea, decaffeinated coffee without sugar, or   just plain water.

Lunch calories: 550.

Dinner:

Kabob: 4 ounces of fat-free steak cut along the grain into 1/4 inch slices. Coat steak slices with 1/4 cup of teriyaki sauce and hot pepper sauce. Cover and marinate in the refrigerator for 30 minutes. Drain steak slices of marinade, reserving marinade. Using   metal skewers, thread steak slices alternating with sweet pepper   chunks and green onion pieces. Brush with marinade while   grilling over medium coals for 3-5 minutes or until Kabobs are slightly pink in center. Serve Kabobs with 1 cup of salad greens   and 1/2 cup of sugar-free ice cream or 1 cup of grapefruit or   orange juice.

Dinner calories: 600.

Day 15: Sunday

Breakfast:

Bacon: 4 slices Boar's head Domestic (140 Cal) + 2 slices of 100% whole-wheat or oat bran toasted bread (170 Cal) + 3 slices of tomatoes (70 Cal) + 1 fistful of your favorite fruit (70-80 cal). Take 1 cup of green tea, decaffeinated coffee without sugar, or just plain water.

Breakfast calories: 450.

Lunch:

Cobb Salad: 1 slice of each of turkey (ham) and Swiss cheese with whites of two hard-boiled eggs and 1 teaspoon of olive oil as a dressing (280 cal) + 1 yogurt Dannon La Creme-4 ounces (140 Cal) +1 cup of grapefruit or orange juice w/pulp (130).

Take 1 cup of green tea, decaffeinated coffee without sugar, or just plain water.

Lunch calories: 550.

Dinner:

Veggie: cook 2 cloves (minced) garlic and1/2 onion (chopped) in olive oil until tender. Stir in 1/4 cup blgur,1/4 cup soybeans, 1/4 cup orange juice, 1/4 cup of vegetable broth (or chicken broth), 1/2 medium carrot, and 1/2 stalk of celery. Bring to boil, reduce heat. Simmer, covered, for 10-12 minutes or until soybeans are tender and liquid is absorbed (470 cal).

Dessert: 1 cup of grapefruit or orange juice with pulp (130 cal). Take 1 cup of green tea and plenty of water.

Dinner calories: 600.

Chapter 14

Healthy Recipes for Life

"HAD WE BUT WORLD ENOUGH, AND TIME—

ANDREW MARVEL

"TO HIS COY MISTRESS,"1681

Breakfast

Apple Oatmeal

Calories: 125 per serving

Ingredients:

1 cup of water; 2 tablespoons grapefruit (or orange) juice concentrate; 1/2 sliced firm banana; 1/4 cup of dried raisins; 1/4 tablespoon of ground cinnamon; 2/3 cup quick-cooking oats; 1/2 cup unpeeled tart apple, chopped; and 1/4 cup oat bran.

1) Combine water, grapefruit, apple, banana, cinnamon, and raisins.

2) Bring to boiling; stir in oats and oat bran.

3) Cook for 1-2 minutes, stirring occasionally; season to taste and serve. (4 servings)

Spinach-filled Omelets

Calories: 125 per serving

Ingredients:

3 whole eggs and 4 egg-whites; 1 tablespoon of canola oil;1/2 cup reduced-fat sharp cheddar cheese, shredded; 1 cup fresh spinach leaves, torn; 1 tablespoon snipped fresh chives; and 1 teaspoon of red pepper relish.

1) Combine eggs, chives, and ground red pepper; beat until frothy.

2) Pour into hot canola oil in a skillet; cook over medium heat.

3) When eggs are set but still shiny, sprinkle with cheese; top with spinach and red pepper relish.

4) Fold one side of omelet partially over filling and top with the remaining spinach and the relish; serve in warm platter. (4 servings)

Rice Cereal

Calories: 125 per serving

Ingredients:

1 cup instant brown rice; 1 cup of 2% A& D fortified milk; 1 1/2 cups of water; dash of nutmeg; and 1/2 cup of any dried fruit (raisins, fig, or plums), chopped.

1) Stir in brown rice in boiling water; reduce heat and simmer, covered, for 5 minutes.

2) Stir in dried fruits; simmer, covered, until rice is tender and liquid is absorbed.

3) Stir in milk and nutmeg; heat through and spoon into bowls.

4) Season to taste with salt and pepper, if desired. (4 servings)

Coffee Cake

Calories: 125 per serving

Ingredients:

1/2 cup all-purpose flour; 1/4 cup honey; 1/2 teaspoon baking powder; 1/2 teaspoon baking soda; 1/4 teaspoon nutmeg; 3 egg-whites; 1/2 cup plain fat-free yogurt; 2 tablespoons of olive (or canola) oil; 1/2 teaspoon vanilla; 1 medium mango (or peaches, nectarines), seeded, peeled, and finely chopped; and 1 tablespoon flaked coconut.

1) Stir together the flour, baking powder, honey, baking soda, and nutmeg; set aside.

2) Stir together the egg whites, yogurt, vanilla, and oil; add to the flour mix.

3) Toss chopped mango with 1 teaspoon of flour; gently fold into batter and spread the batter into the prepared baking pan.

4) Sprinkle with coconut and bake at 350⁰ F for 30- 40 minutes or until a wooden toothpick inserted near center comes out clean; serve warm. (4 servings)

SOUPS

Wild Rice Soup

Calories: 250 per serving (1 cup)

Ingredients:

2 14.5 -ounce cans chicken broth, 4 cloves garlic, minced; 3 cups of chopped tomatoes; 1 9-ounce- package frozen chopped cooked chicken breast; 1 cup of zucchini, finely chopped; 1 teaspoon thyme, dried and crushed; and 6.2 - ounce package quick-cooking wild rice.

1) Combine the chicken broth, garlic, and thyme; bring to boiling.

2) Stir in tomatoes, zucchini, and chicken; return to boiling.

3) Reduce heat; simmer, covered, for 6 minutes.

4) Stir in cooked wild rice.

5) Let stand for 5 minutes and serve. (Makes 4 servings)

Lentil Soup

Calories: 100 per serving (1 cup)

Ingredients:

1 small onion, chopped; 1/2 cup dried lentils; 1 bell pepper, chopped; 1 carrot, chopped, 4 garlic cloves, minced; 2 bay leaves; 2 teaspoons of olive oil; 1 quart (4 cups) water; 1 tablespoon balsamic vinegar; and 1/2 can (14 ounces) un-drained, crushed tomatoes.

1) Heat olive oil in a saucepan over medium-high heat and cook onion with stirring occasionally.

2) Stir in carrot, bell pepper, and garlic; cook for 3 minutes. Stir in the remaining ingredients and bring to boil.

3) Reduce heat; simmer uncovered 15- 20 minutes (until lentils are tender).

4) Remove bay leaves, season to taste with salt and pepper, and serve. (4 servings)

Garbanzo Soup

Calories: 200 calories per serving (1 cup)

3/4 cup dry garbanzo beans; 2 cups sliced carrots; 1 medium onion, chopped; 3 cups of water; 1 cup fresh spinach, shredded; 2 teaspoons instants chicken bouillon granules; 2 teaspoons of crushed thyme; 1 cup sliced celery; and 3/4 pounds skinless, boneless chicken breast halves.

1) Cover beans in a pan with water enough to cover by 2 inches and bring to boil; reduce heat and simmer, uncovered, for 10 minutes.

2) Remove from heat, cover, and let stand for 1 hour. Drain and rinse beans.

3) Place beans, chicken, carrots, onion, thyme, and bouillon granules in 3 cups of water; cover and cook on medium heat for 12- 15 minutes.

4) Remove the chicken; cool slightly.

5) Cut the chicken into bite size pieces and return to pan.

6) Stir in the shredded spinach and thyme; boil for 2 minutes.

7) Let stand for 5 minutes and serve. (4 servings)

Vegetable Soup

Calories: 250 per serving (1 cup)

Ingredients:

1 large onion, chopped; 2 stalks of celery, chopped; 6 cloves of garlic, minced; 3 large carrots, chopped; 1 tablespoon of olive oil; 1/4 teaspoon of dried thyme; and 1/4 cup of mushroom pieces.

1) Place the olive oil, carrots, celery, and onion in a nonstick pan; toss to coat with olive oil and bake in oven for 12 minutes at 450⁰ F.

2) Remove the pan from oven, add 1 cup of water and stir to lessen vegetables.

3) Pour Pan's ingredients with the remaining ingredients into a pot and bring to boiling; reduce heat, cover, and simmer for 30 minutes at medium heat.

4) Let stand for 5 minutes, season with salt and pepper to taste, and serve. (4 servings)

Shrimp Soup

Calories: 200 per serving () 1 cup)

Ingredients:

2 medium-cucumber, chopped; 1/2 cup of chopped onion; 2 tablespoon olive oil; 2 cloves of garlic, minced; 1 8-ounce package frozen peeled, cooked shrimp, thawed; 1 medium red pepper, chopped; 1 tablespoon fresh cilantro; 2 tablespoon red wine (or vinegar); 1/2 cup clam juice; 1 cup vegetable juice; and 6 large tomatoes, chopped.

1) Combine all the ingredients in a large bowl and cover.

2) Refrigerate for 6- 24 hours to blend favors.

3) Ladle into soup bowls; season to taste with salt and pepper. (4 servings)

Red Bean Soup

Calories: 250 per serving (1 cup)

Ingredients:

1/2 cup red beans, dried; 4 medium tomatoes, diced; 1 tablespoon olive oil; 1 large onion, chopped; 5 cloves garlic, minced; 4 cups of water; and 1/2 package (6 ounces) baked, pressed tofu, diced.

1) Soak beans in cold water for 4-6 hours; drain.

2) In a pot, sauté onions, and garlic in olive oil until soft.

3) Add the red beans and water, cover; bring to boiling.

4) Reduce heat, add minced tomatoes, and simmer until desired tenderness.

5) Add tofu, season to taste with salt and pepper.

6) Let it stand for 5 minutes and serve. (4 servings)

Goulash Soup

Calories: 250 per serving (1 cup)

Ingredients:

2 14.5- ounce can minced tomatoes, un-drained; 12 ounces boneless, fat-free beef sirloin steak; 1 tablespoon olive oil; 2 medium onions, coarsely chopped; 3 cups of water; 1 cup chopped carrot; 2 cloves garlic, minced; 2 cups cabbage, sliced; 1 teaspoon unsweetened cocoa powder; 2 14.5 -ounce can beef broth; 1 cup of dried noodles; 2 teaspoons paprika; and 1/2 cup of fat-free dairy sour cream.

1) Cut Steak into 1/2-inch cubes and add to olive oil in a large saucepan.

2) Cook and stir for 3- 5 minutes or until meat is brown.

3) Add onion and stir for 3-5 minutes or until onion is tender.

4) Stir in water, beef broth, un-drained tomatoes, carrot, garlic, and cocoa powder.

5) Bring to boiling; reduce heat.

6) Simmer, uncovered, about 15-20 minutes or until the meat is tender.

7) Stir in noodles, cabbage, and paprika.

8) Simmer, uncovered, for 5-8 minutes more or until noodles are tender.

9) Remove from heat; stir in sour cream.

10) Let it stand for 5 minutes and serve. (4 servings)

Teriyaki Soup

Calories: 250 per serving (1 cup)

8 ounces boneless beef sirloin steak; 3 cups water; 1/2 cup uncooked long rice; 1 teaspoon instant beef bouillon granules; 2 cups small broccoli flowerets; 2 tablespoons light teriyaki sauce; 1 tablespoon grated ginger; 2 large carrots, cut into bite-size; 1 cup apple juice; 1 large onion, sliced; and 3 teaspoon olive or canola oil.

1) In a sauce pan, heat olive (or canola) oil over medium-high heat and add meat, onion.

2) Cook and stir for 3-6 minutes or until meat is brown; remove meat mixture and set aside.

3) In the same saucepan, combine water, carrots, rice, ginger, bouillon granules, apple juice, and water; bring to boiling.

4) Reduce heat; simmer, covered, for 12-15 minutes or until carrots are tender.

5) Stir in the meat mixture and broccoli; simmer, covered, for 3-5 minutes.

6) Stir in the teriyaki sauce; ladle into soup bowls. (4 servings)

Black Bean Soup

Calories: 250 per serving (1 cup)

Ingredients:

1 large onion, chopped; 5 cloves garlic, sliced; 2 carrots, chopped; 2 tablespoon olive (or canola) oil; 2 stalks celery, chopped; 8 cups of vegetable broth; 2 15ounce-cans of black beans, rinsed and drained; 1 teaspoon ground coriander; 1 tablespoon balsamic vinegar; and 1 bunch cilantro leaves, chopped.

1) Heat oil in a saucepan over medium-high heat; add onion and cook for 5 minutes, with stirring occasionally.

2) Add carrot, celery, and garlic; cook until soft, about 4-6 minutes.

3) add vegetable broth, beans, and coriander; simmer, uncovered, for 8 minutes.

4) Stir in vinegar and blend (food processor) to desired consistency.

5) Ladle into soup bowls; season with salt and pepper. (4 servings)

Creamy Tomato Soup

Calories: 250 per serving (1 cup)

Ingredients:

2 14.5 -ounce can tomato, diced, un-drained; 2 10.5- ounce condensed tomato soup, undiluted; 1 tablespoon olive (or canola) oil; 2 cups of 2% A& D fortified milk; 1 teaspoon of dried basil; 5 clove garlic, minced; 1 large onion (or shallot), chopped; 1 teaspoon of paprika; and 8 ounces of Swiss cheese, cubed or sliced.

1) Sauté onion in oil until tender; stir in tomatoes, soup, milk, basil, paprika, and garlic; bring to boiling.

2) Reduce heat; cover and simmer for 10 minutes.

3) Stir in cheese until melted.

4) Season to taste and serve immediately in soup bowls. (4 serving)

Zucchini Beef Soup

Calories: 250 per serving (1 cup)

Ingredients:

16 ounces of ground beef; 4 celery ribs, thinly sliced; 1 cup of chopped onion, 1 cup of chopped green or yellow pepper; 2 28-ounce cans of tomato, diced, un-drained; 6 medium zucchini, cubed; 4 cups of water; 1 tablespoon of Italian seasoning; 1 tablespoon of beef bouillon granules,; and 2 slices of Parmesan cheese, shredded.

1) Cook beef, celery, onion, and pepper over medium-high heat in a saucepan until meat is no longer pink and vegetables are tender; drain.

2) Stir in the tomatoes, zucchini, Italian seasoning, bouillon, and water. Bring to boiling.

3) Reduce heat; cover and simmer for 20-25 minutes or until zucchini is tender; garnish with Parmesan cheese.

4) Season to taste with salt and black pepper; ladle into soup bowls. (4 servings)

Turkey Soup

Calories: 250 per serving) 1 cup)

Ingredients:

1/2 cup Celery, chopped; 1 medium onion, chopped; 2 tablespoons of olive (or canola) oil; 6 ounces of chicken-flavored ramen noodles; 2 10.5 ounce cans of condensed turkey noodle soup, undiluted; 2 cups of chicken broth; and 1 cup of cubed cooked turkey.

1) Sauté celery and onion in olive oil until tender.

2) Stir noodles, water, soup, broth, turkey, and pepper into celery mixture; do not use seasoning packet from ramen noodles.

4) Cook for 3-5 minutes or until noodles are tender and heated through.

5) Season to taste with salt and pepper; ladle into soup bowls. (4 servings)

Fiesta Soup

Calories: 250 per serving (1 cup)

Ingredients:

2 10.5 ounce cans of diced tomatoes and green chilies; 1 can (15.5 ounces) whole kernel corn, drained; 1 can (15 ounces) black beans, rinsed and drained; 2 slices of Parmesan, shredded; and 1/4 cup of sour cream.

1) Combine tomatoes, corn, and beans in a saucepan; heat through.

2) Garnish servings with Parmesan cheese and sour cream.

3) Season to taste with salt and pepper; ladle into soup bowls (4 servings)

Roast Pork Soup

Calories: 250 per serving (1 cup)

Ingredients:

3 cups cubed cooked pork roast; 1 medium potato, peeled and chopped; 1 large onion, chopped; 1 can (15 ounces) navy beans, rinsed and drained; 1 can (14.5 ounces) Italian diced tomatoes, un-drained; 4 cups of water; and 1 teaspoon of minced basil.

1) Combine all ingredients except basil in a saucepan; bring to boiling.

2) Reduce heat; cover and simmer for 40 minutes or until vegetables are crisp-tender.

3) Sprinkle with basil and salt to taste; ladle into soup bowls. (4 servings)

Chicken Rice Soup

Calories: 250 per serving (1 cup)

Ingredients:

6 cups of chicken broth; 3 cups of cubed cooked chicken; 4 celery ribs, chopped; 3 medium carrots, chopped; 2 medium green or yellow pepper, chopped; 2 medium onions (or shallot), chopped; 1/2 cup uncooked wild rice; 1 teaspoon of minced fresh cilantro pr parsley; 1 teaspoon of oregano; and 1/2 teaspoon of ground cumin.

1) Combine all ingredients in a saucepan and bring to boiling; reduce heat.

2) Cover and simmer for 20-25 minutes or until rice and vegetables are tender.

3) Ladle into soup bowls; season to taste with salt and pepper. (4 serving)

SALAD

Cabbage Salad

Calories: 250 per serving

Ingredients:

8 cups of cabbage, shredded; 2 medium bananas, diced, 1 cup pecan, chopped; 2 medium red apples, diced; 2 tablespoon virgin olive; 1/2 cup of 2% A& D fortified milk; 4 tablespoon raisins; and 2 tablespoon lemon juice.

1) Combine the cabbage, apples, bananas, and raisins in a bowl; set aside.

2) In a jar with a tight-fitting lid, combine milk and lemon juice and salt if desired; shake well.

3) Pour over cabbage mixture and toss to coat with virgin olive. (4 servings)

Middle Eastern Salad

Calories: 250 per serving

Ingredients:

2 medium tomatoes, diced; 2 scallions, chopped; 2 yellow pepper, chopped; 12 black olives, pitted and chopped; 2 cucumber, diced; 1/4 cup of lemon juice; 1/4 cup of virgin oil; and 1/4 cup of feta cheese, crumbled.

1) Combine all ingredients in a bowl; season to taste with salt and pepper, and serve. (4 servings)

Pork Salad

Calories: 250 per serving

Ingredients:

16 ounces of pork loin chops, cut 3/4 inch thick; 5 slices turkey bacon; 1 teaspoon honey; 2 large apples, coarsely chopped; 1 teaspoon of back pepper, 1 tablespoon nutmeg; 6 cups of cabbage and carrot mix, sliced; 3/4 cup cider vinegar;3/4 cup apple juice; and 1 tablespoon caraway seed.

1) Sprinkle pork chops with pepper and nutmeg; broil for 6- 8 minutes or until pork is slightly pink in center and juices run clear.

2) Combine cabbage and apple in another bowl; set aside.

3) In a medium skillet, cook bacon over medium heat until crisp; drain and crumble bacon.

4) Combine vinegar, apple juice, honey and caraway seed; bring to boiling.

5) Pour over cabbage mixture; add bacon and toss gently to coat.

6) Arrange pork slices on top the salad serving. (4 servings)

Japanese Salad

Calories: 250 per serving

Ingredients:

Part A: 4 tablespoon olive oil; 4 tablespoon rice vinegar; 1/2 medium onion (or shallot), chopped; 1 large carrot, chopped; 1 tablespoon grated ginger; and 1/2 teaspoon soy sauce.

Part B: 1 large head romaine lettuce, shredded; 1/2 cup fresh bean sprouts; and 1 tablespoon pumpkin seed

1) Combine part A and blend in food processor; puree until smooth.

2) Toss lettuce with part A; top with bean sprouts and pumpkin seeds.

3) Season to taste with salt and pepper; serve. (4 servings)

Caesar Salad

Calories: 250 per serving

Ingredients:

3/4 cup Parmesan cheese, shredded; 6 cups torn romaine; 1/2 cup 2% A&D fortified Milk; 3 tablespoons olive oil; 2 tablespoons lemon juice; 1 cup seasoned crotons; 2 cups cherry tomato, halved; and 2 cloves of garlic, minced.

1) Combine the milk, 1/2 cup of parmesan cheese, lemon juice and milk; mix well.

2) Add the romaine and the remaining Parmesan.

3) Just before serving, dress with olive oil and toss to coat.

4) Top with croutons and cherry tomatoes, if desired; serve. (4 serving)

Millet Salad

Calories: 250 per serving

Ingredients:

3 tablespoons olive oil; 1/2 cup millet; 2 cups shrimp, peeled, deveined and cooked; 4 ounces of chestnut, sliced and drained; 1/2 cup red onion, chopped; 1/2 cup rice vinegar; 1 tablespoon orange peel, finely shredded; 1 teaspoon toasted sesame seeds; 1/4 cup snipped fresh cilantro; 1 medium mango, seeded, peeled, and chopped; and 2 cups of water.

1) Cook millet in 1 tablespoon of olive oil with occasional stirring for 2 minutes; carefully add the water.

2) Bring to boiling, reduce heat; simmer, covered, about 25 minutes or until millet is fluffy and water is absorbed.

3) Transfer millet to a large bowl; add shrimp, mango, water chestnut, onion, and cilantro.

4) Toss gently to combine; dress with olive oil, vinegar, orange peel, and sesame seed.

5) Season to taste with salt and black pepper; serve. (4 servings)

Turkish Salad

Calories: 250 per serving

Ingredients:

2 pounds of fresh spinach; 8 cherry tomatoes, halved; 12 scallions, thinly sliced; 3 tablespoons olive oil; 2 cups of plain, nonfat yogurt; 3 cloves of garlic, minced; and 1/2 teaspoon dried thyme.

1) Combine spinach, tomatoes, and scallions in a bowl.

2) Combine the yogurt, minced garlic, and yogurt; mix well.

3) Season to taste with salt and black pepper; toss with olive oil to coat and serve (4 servings)

Cashew Salad

Calories: 250 per serving

Ingredients:

3 tablespoons of olive oil; 5 tablespoons of grapefruit juice; 2 tablespoons of rice wine vinegar; 2 teaspoons of grated fresh gingerroot; 2 teaspoons of soy sauce; 1 teaspoon of sesame oil; 4 cups of shredded lettuce; 1 cup of sliced cucumber; 2 bunches of chopped cilantro; 1 cup of shredded carrot; 5 tablespoons of cashew; and 1/2 cup of chopped green onion.

1) Combine all ingredients except cashew and green onion.

2) Season to taste with salt and black pepper; top plates with cashew and green onion and serve. (4 servings)

Dijon Salad

Calories: 250 per serving

Ingredients:

1 cup olive oil; 3 tablespoons lemon juice; 3 garlic cloves, minced; 2 teaspoons Dijon mustard; 7 cups of torn romaine; 1/4 cup of grated Parmesan cheese; 1/2 cup of red onion, sliced; and 1 cup of salad croutons.

1) Dressing: combine oil, lemon juice, garlic, and mustard; mix well.

2) Combine romaine and cheese; drizzle with dressing.

3) Toss to coat; top with croutons and green onions, and serve. (4 servings)

Fruit Salad

Calories: 250 per serving

Ingredients:

2 tablespoons of olive oil; 2 medium cucumber, peeled, seeded and diced; 2 medium tart apple, chopped; 1 cup of mango, seeded and sliced; 1 cup of red seedless grapes; 1/2 cup sour cream; 1/2 cup of chopped almonds; and 1 tablespoon of fresh parsley, minced.

1) Combine the cucumber, apple, mango and grapes.

2) Combine the sour cream and parsley; pour over cucumber mixture and toss to coat.

3) Dress with olive oil and top with chopped almonds; serve. (4 servings)

Beet Salad

Calories: 250 per serving

Ingredients:

4 cups of beets; 1/2 cup of rice or cider vinegar; 4 tablespoons of olive oil; 2 teaspoons of wasabi powder (Japanese horseradish); and 2 large onions, chopped.

1) Boil the beets in water over medium heat until tender; drain.

2) Thinly slice the beets and combine with other ingredients.

3) Dress with olive oil; season to taste and serve. (4 servings)

Macaroni Salad

Calories: 250 per serving

Ingredients:

16 ounces of elbow macaroni; 1 1/2 cup of green pepper, diced; 1 cup of sweet pickle relish; 4 ounces of diced pimientos, drained; 2 table spoons of chopped onion; 1 cup of sour cream; and 1/2 cup of 2% A&D fortified milk.

1) Cook macaroni until tender; rinse in cold water and drain.

2) Combine macaroni, green pepper, pickle relish, pimientos and onion.

3) In a small bowl combine the remaining ingredients; mix well.

4) Pour over macaroni and toss to coat; season to taste and serve. (4 servings)

Salmon Salad

Calories: 250 per serving

Ingredients:

1 cup of canned salmon, cut into 1/2 inch thick; 12 cherry tomatoes, halved; 1/4 cup reduced-sodium soy sauce; 1/4 cup olive oil; 1/2 teaspoon toasted sesame oil (seed); 1 tablespoon lemon juice; and 2 cups of shredded salad greens of your choice.

1) Combine all ingredients except cherry tomatoes in a large bowl; mix well.

2) Dress with olive oil and top with cherry tomatoes; season to taste and serve. (4 servings)

Grapefruit Salad

Calories: 250 per serving

Ingredients:

2 large bunches of spinach washed and trimmed; 1/2 cup almond, roasted and halved; 2 grapefruit, sectioned; 4 green onions, chopped; 2 tablespoons olive oil; 2 tablespoons red wine; and 2 teaspoon honey.

1) Combine all ingredients except grapefruits and green onions; mix well.

2) Top plates with grapefruit sections and green onion slices; season to taste with salt and black pepper. (4 servings)

Mediterranean Salad

Calories: 250 per serving

Ingredients:

10 ounces of boneless lamb sirloin chops, cut into 1/2 inch thick; 2 cups of spinach, torn; 1 cup of canned garbanzo beans, rinsed and drained; 1/4 cup of green onion, chopped; 2 cloves of garlic, minced; 1/2 cup of nonfat, plain yogurt; 1/4 cup of dried golden raisins; 1/4 cup of cucumber, seeded and chopped; 2 teaspoons of snipped fresh rosemary, dried and crushed; and 1 tablespoon of olive oil.

1) Rub rosemary and garlic over fat-trimmed lamb chops; broil chops until slightly pink in center.

2) In a large bowl, toss the spinach, garbanzo beans, and cucumber.

3) Top plates with lamb slices over spinach mixture.

4) In a small bowl combine yogurt, olive oil; and green onion; pour over salad plates.

5) Dress plates with olive oil and season to taste; serve. (4 servings)

Kiwifruit Salad

Calories: 250 per serving

Ingredients:

6 cups of salad greens (any greens of your choice); 2 medium red apples, diced; 1 cup of unsweetened raspberries, 1 cup of unsweetened blueberries; 6 kiwifruits, peeled and sliced; 3 tablespoons of olive oil; and 2 cups of poppy seed.

1) Toss the salad greens, onion, and fruits; drizzle with poppy seeds.

2) Dress with olive oil and season to taste with salt and pepper; serve. (4 servings)

Kiwifruit or passion fruit works fine.

Broccoli Salad

Calories: 250 per serving

Ingredients:

4 cups broccoli florets; 3 cups of cooked shrimp, deveined and peeled; 4 medium carrots, thinly sliced; 4 small onions, sliced and separated into rings; 5 ounces of sliced black olives, drained; 4 ounces of pimientos, drained; 1/2 cup honey; 1 1/2 cups of chopped almonds; and 8 ounces of nonfat- Italian salad dressing.

1) Combine broccoli, carrots, onions, olives, cooked shrimp, and pimientos; add honey and dressing and toss to coat.

2) Cover and refrigerate of at least 4 hours, stirring occasionally.

3) Just before serving, stir in chopped almonds; serve. (4 servings)

Ranch Salad

Calories: 250 per serving

Ingredients:

16 ounces of boneless beef top sirloin steak, cut 3/4 inch thick; 2 tablespoons lemon juice; 1 tablespoon of olive oil; 2 cloves garlic, minced; 4 cups of torn salad greens (of your choice); 1 cup of carrot, peeled and thinly sliced; 1/2 cup thinly sliced radishes; 1/2 cup of red onion; and 1/2 cup bottled fat-free ranch salad dressing.

1) Cook the red onions in olive oil over medium-high heat for 2 minutes or until browned, stirring occasionally; set aside.

2) Sprinkle fat-trimmed steak with lemon juice and garlic; rub in with your fingers.

3) Cook steak over medium heat until desired doneness, turning once.

4) Toss together the salad greens, carrots, and radishes.

5) Arrange steak strips over greens mixture; drizzle with ranch dressing and sprinkle with fried red onions. (4 servings)

Meatless

Chinese Veggie

Calories: 250 per serving

Ingredients:

8 ounces dried pasta; 1 tablespoons dark, roasted sesame oil; 1 tablespoon olive oil; 6 ounces baked, pressed tofu, cut into 1/2-inch cubes; 4 tablespoons rice wine vinegar; 1 teaspoon hot pepper flakes; 3 cups of broccoli florets; and 3 tablespoons garlic, minced.

1) Cook the broccoli until tender, about 4-5 minutes; remove, rinse and drain.

2) Cook the pasta in boiling water and drain.

3) Stir -fry garlic and red pepper in olive and olive oil in a skillet for 20 seconds; add the broccoli, tofu cubes, and soy sauce; stir-fry for 40 seconds and remove from heat.

4) Toss the pasta with the broccoli mixture; season to taste with salt and serve warm or at room temperature. (4 servings)

Japanese Veggie

Calories: 250 per serving

Ingredients:

2 cups of mushroom, halved; 1 cup of broccoli florets; 1/2 red bell pepper; 6 ounces of baked tofu, cubed; 2 green opinions, chopped; 1 teaspoon soy sauce; 2 garlic cloves, sliced; 1/2 red onion, sliced; 1 tablespoon olive oil; 1 tablespoon sesame oil; and 1 teaspoon sesame seeds.

1) Stir-fry onion and garlic in olive, sesame oil and pepper flakes for 2 minutes in a large skillet.

2) Stir-fry broccoli, red pepper, mushrooms, and soy sauce until vegetables are crisp-tender or for 2-3 minutes.

3) Add tofu, green onions, and sesame seeds; stir-fry until heated through.

4) Season to taste with salt and serve warm or at room temperature. (4 servings)

Veggie Fiber

Calories: 250 per serving

Ingredients:

1 1/2 cups of dry red lentils, rinsed and drained; 2 medium red onions, chopped; 2 tablespoon olive oil; 1 medium yellow or green sweet pepper, cut into 1/2- inch rings; 5 cups of water; and 1 teaspoon snipped fresh thyme.

1) Stir-fry onions until browned, stirring occasionally.

2) Add pepper and thyme and stir for 2 minutes.

3) Add the water and lentils; bring to boiling, reduce heat, simmer for 15-20 minutes.

4) Season to taste with salt and pepper; serve. (4 servings)

Basil Pasta

Calories: 250 per serving

Ingredients:

2 cups of uncooked pasta; 1 medium onion, chopped; 2 tablespoons of olive oil; 2 tablespoons of dried basil; 4 ounces (1 cup) of Parmesan cheese.

1) Cook the pasta in water until tender and drain.

2) Sauté onion in olive oil until browned; stir in dried basil for 1 minute.

3) Add pasta to basil mixture; remove from heat and stir in cheese just until begins to melt,

4) Season to taste with salt and pepper; serve warm or at room temperature. (4 servings)

Soybean Pilaf

Calories: 250 per serving

Ingredients:

3/4 cup of soybeans; 1/2 cup of bulgur; 1 medium onion, chopped; 2 cloves garlic, minced; 2 tablespoons olive oil; 1 cup of orange juice; 1 cup of vegetable broth; 1 medium carrot, cut into thin bite-size strips; 1/2 stalk celery, sliced; and 2 grapefruits, sectioned.

1) Stir-fry onion in olive oil until tender.

2) Stir in bulgur, soybeans, orange juice, carrot, and celery; bring to boiling, reduce heat.

3) Simmer, covered, until soybeans are tender and liquid is absorbed.

4) Stir in grapefruits; season to taste and serve. (4 servings)

Veggie Puree

Calories: 250 per serving

Ingredients:

12 ounces of fresh spinach, chopped; 3 tablespoons roasted cashew, chopped; 1 tablespoon olive oil; 1 onion, thinly sliced; 5 cloves of garlic, minced; 1/2 cup water; 1 tablespoon fresh ginger, minced; and 1 tablespoon curry powder.

1) Blend cashew until fine, add water; blend for 2 minutes.

2) Cook the garlic and ginger in olive oil until tender; stir in spinach and curry powder, reduce heat to low and add cashew.

3) Simmer, covered, for 15-20 minutes; remove from heat, let cool slightly, and process (food processor) until smooth.

4) Pour the puree into garlic mixture and heat through.

5) Season to taste with salt and pepper; serve. (4 servings)

Italian Veggie

Calories: 250 per serving

Ingredients:

12 ounces of pasta, cooked; 1 can (15 ounces) of northern beans, rinsed and drained; 2 celery ribs, sliced; 1 medium onion, chopped; 1 jar (14 ounces) spaghetti sauce; and 2 cans (14 ounces each) stewed, diced tomatoes.

Seasonings:

1/4 teaspoon garlic salt; 1/4 teaspoon dried basil; and 1/4 teaspoon dried parsley flakes.

1) Combine the tomatoes, beans, spaghetti sauce, celery, onion and seasonings.

2) Bring to boiling and reduce heat; simmer for 20 minutes or until vegetables are tender.

3) Serve over hot pasta. (4 servings)

Tarragon Green Beans

Calories: 250 per serving

Ingredients:

8 cups of frozen cut green beans; 1 large onion, chopped; 1 celery rib, chopped; 3 tablespoons of olive oil; 1 cup of apple cider; 3/4 teaspoon dried tarragon; and 1 cup of finely chopped green pepper.

1) Combine the beans and water; bring to boiling and drain.

2) Reduce heat; cover and simmer for 15 minutes or until tender.

3) Sauté the onion, celery and green pepper in olive oil until tender; stir in tarragon and apple cider.

4) Add the sauté mixture into the beans mixture and toss to coat.

5) Season to taste with salt and black pepper; serve. (4 servings)

Mediterranean Veggie

Calories: 250 per serving

Ingredients:

1 cup of brown rice; 2 cups of eggplant, cut into 3/4 -inch cubes; 1 cup of zucchini, sliced 1/2 inch thick; 6 cloves of garlic, minced; 1 can (15 ounces) kidney beans, rinsed and drained; 2 large tomatoes, chopped; 1 tablespoon balsamic vinegar; 2 teaspoons of basil; 5 cups of water; 1 medium onion, chopped; and 2 tablespoons of olive oil.

1) Stir-fry garlic and onion in olive oil until onions are tender; stir in tomato and basil and heat through.

2) Combine rice, water, eggplant, zucchini, and garlic with onion mixture in a large pan; cook and stir until rice is tender.

3) Stir in beans; simmer, uncovered, for 5 minutes or until beans are tender.

4) Stir in vinegar; ladle the vegetable mixture into bowls, and season to taste with salt and black pepper. (4 servings)

Couscous

Calories: 250 per serving

Ingredients:

3 cups of boiling water; 1 cup whole-wheat couscous; 1 teaspoon canola oil; 1 medium tomato, chopped; 1 tablespoon fresh parsley leaves, chopped; 2 cloves of garlic, minced; 4 tablespoons of cashews, toasted.

1) Pour couscous in hot water and stir; let stand for 15 minutes.

2) Loosen the couscous with a fork, stir in canola oil, and add the rest of ingredients.

3) Season to taste with salt and serve. (4 servings)

Fish and Seafood

Grapefruit Swordfish

Calories: 250 per serving

Ingredients:

16 ounces of fresh or frozen swordfish steak, cut into 1 -inch thick; 1/2 cup of grapefruit juice; 6 tablespoons of unsweetened apple cider; 2 tablespoons of Dijon mustard; 1 tablespoon of soy sauce; and 4 ounces of dried pasta.

1) Thaw fish, if frozen; rinse, pat dry with paper towels and put inside a plastic bag.

2) For marinade, combine grapefruit juice, mustard, apple cider, and soy sauce.

3) Pour marinade over fish; seal the plastic bag; marinate in the refrigerator for 1 to 2 hours, turning bag occasionally.

4) Drain fish, reserving marinade; grill fish over medium coals for 10 to 12 minutes or until fish flakes easily when tested with a fork, brushing with some marinade halfway through grilling.

5) Cook pasta until tender; drain.

6) Toss the pasta with the heated rest of the marinade; serve with fish. (4 servings)

Mediterranean Steak

Calories: 250 per serving

Ingredients:

2 pounds of tuna steak, cut into 1-inch thick; 2 tablespoons of olive oil; 2 medium tomatoes, finely diced; 10 green olives, pitted and diced; 2 tablespoons scallions, chopped; 3 cloves garlic, minced; and a pinch of dried oregano.

1) Rinse the tuna steaks and pat dry with paper towels; brush them with olive oil.

2) Marinade: mix all other ingredients and set aside.

3) Grill the steaks or broil until desired doneness.

4) Cover the steaks with the marinade mixture, and serve cold or hot. (4 servings)

Mango- Red Snapper

Calories: 250 per serving

Ingredients:

1 1/4 pound of fresh or frozen skinless red snapper fillets, cut into 1/2 - inch thick; 1 medium onion, finely chopped; 1 cup of peeled and chopped mango; 3 tablespoons of olive oil; 4 lime wedges; 2 teaspoons of cornstarch; and a pinch of red pepper.

1) Thaw the fish, if frozen; rinse and pat dry with paper towels.

2) Sprinkle the fish with a pitch of red pepper; set aside.

3) Sauce: cook onion in olive oil until tender; stir in cornstarch and some crushed pepper.

4) Cook and stir until thickened and blobby; add mango and cook, with stirring occasionally, for 2 minutes.

5) Remove from heat, cover and keep warm.

6) Cook the fish in olive oil until fish flakes easily when tested with a fork, turning gently once during cooking.

7) Spoon the sauce over fish; serve with lime wedges. (4 servings)

Poached Salmon

Calories: 250 per serving

Ingredients:

1 1/2 pound of salmon fillet; 3 carrots, peeled and sliced; 2 medium onions, chopped; 3 stalks of celery, sliced; 2 tablespoons of lime juice; and 1 cup red wine.

1) Rinse salmon fillet and cut into portions.

2) Broil the salmon, carrots, onion, celery, and red wine, uncovered.

3) Reduce heat and simmer uncovered for 5 more minutes.

4) Serve fish cold or warm; add lemon juice, if desired. (4 servings)

Fried Fish Fillets

Calories: 250 per serving

Ingredients:

24 ounces of fish fillets; 24 ounces of mushrooms; sliced; 5 scallions; thinly sliced; 3 tablespoons of olive oil; and 4 fresh lemon wedges.

1)Cook the fish in olive oil in a skillet until fish flakes easily when tested with a fork, turning once; remove into a plate; sprinkle the scallions on the fish.

2) Add mushrooms into the skillet and cook until browned.

3) Serve fish with mushrooms and lemon wedges; season to taste with salt and black pepper. (4 servings)

Teriyaki Sea Bass

Calories: 250 per serving

Ingredients:

24 ounces of fresh or frozen sea bass fillets, cut into 1-inch; 4 teaspoons of soy sauce; 6 tablespoons of rice wine; 4 tablespoons of sesame seeds, toasted; 3 teaspoons of olive oil; 4 lemon wedges; and 4 teaspoons of honey.

1) Thaw fish, if frozen; rinse and pat dry with paper towels.

2) Glaze sauce: combine soy sauce, rice wine, and honey; bring to boiling and reduce heat.

3) Simmer, uncovered, until the glaze is reduced to about 1/4 cup.

4) In a large skillet, cook the fish in olive oil for 8 to 12 minutes or until fish flakes easily when tested with a fork, gently turning once.

5) Drizzle the glaze sauce over the fish and sprinkle with sesame seeds. Serve with lemon wedges and season to taste with salt and black pepper. (4 servings)

Poultry

Mediterranean Chicken

Calories: 250 per serving

Ingredients:

Chicken ingredients: 4 skinless chicken breast halves; 1 medium tomato, chopped; 1 medium tomato, chopped; 8 green olives, pitted and halved; 1 teaspoon of wine vinegar; 1 tablespoon olive oil.

Soybean ingredients: 16 ounces of soybeans, rinsed and drained; 1 tomato chopped; 3 cloves of garlic, minced; 1 tablespoon of olive oil; 1/4 cup of chopped fresh mixed herbs; and 2 teaspoon of red wine.

1) Place each chicken breast in a resalable, microwave plastic bag; combine remaining chicken ingredients and spoon over each chicken breast.

2) Reseal plastic bags; microwave for 15 minutes or until chicken breasts are cooked through.

3) In a saucepan, cook garlic in olive oil for 2-3 minutes; add remaining ingredients of soybean and cook until heated through.

4) Serve chicken bags and soybeans alongside; season to taste with salt and pepper. (4 servings)

Cornmeal Chicken

Calories: 250 per serving

4 skinless chicken breast halves; 3 tablespoon of olive oil; 1 cup of cornmeal; 4 teaspoons of cumin, ground; 2 teaspoons of onion powder; 2 teaspoons of oregano; and 1/2 teaspoon cayenne pepper.

1) **Coating mixture:** In a re-sealable plastic bag, combine cornmeal, onion, cumin, oregano, and garlic powder; store in a cool place for up to 6 hours.

2) Dip chicken in olive oil and place in a re-sealable microwave plastic bag; coat each with 1/2 cup of the coating mixture and shake to coat.

3) Cook each at microwave for 15 minutes or until juices run clear.

4) Serve packets with salt and pepper. (4 servings)

Tabboulah Kabobs

Calories: 250 per serving

Ingredients:

Chicken Ingredients: 4 skinless chicken breast halves, cut into 1-inch cubes; 1 medium onion, quartered; 1 medium tomato, quartered; 1 green bell pepper, seeded, stemmed and quartered; 4 mushrooms, halved; 1/2 teaspoon of dried sage; and 1 teaspoon of dried oregano.

Tabboulah Ingredients: 1/2 cup of bulgur wheat; 1 1/2 cup of water; 1 tablespoon of olive oil; 2 tablespoons of lemon juice; 1 medium tomato, sliced; 4 green onions, sliced; 1 small bunch fresh mint leaves, finely chopped; and 1 large bunch parsley, finely chopped.

1)Alternate chicken cubes, onion, tomato, bell pepper, and mushrooms onto metal skewers; cook on covered grill 4-6 minutes per side, or until chicken is cooked through and vegetables are tender.

2) Prepare Tabboulah: place bulgur wheat in medium bowl add water; mix well.

3)Let tabboulah mix stand until all water is absorbed, about 30 to 40 minutes; pour off excess water.

4) Add remaining taboulah ingredients and mix well; season to taste with salt and black pepper.

5) Serve tabboulah with grilled chicken and vegetables. (4 servings)

Dijon Chicken

Calories: 250 per serving

Ingredients:

4 skinless chicken breast halves; 2 tablespoons of Dijon mustard; 4 small potatoes, halved; and 2 tablespoons of olive oil.

1) Dip chicken breasts in mustard and cook in olive oil until juices run clear, about 10 minutes; set aside.

2) Sir in potatoes in olive oil and cook until tender.

3) Serve chicken with potatoes; season to taste with salt and pepper. (4 servings)

Caribbean Chicken

Calories: 250 per serving

Ingredients:

4 skinless chicken breast halves; 1 small grapefruit, peeled and quartered; 2 ripe kiwifruits, peeled and quartered; 2 ripe carambola, cut into 1/2-inch slices; 1/2 teaspoon hot paprika; 2 teaspoons of orange peel, finely shredded; 2 ripe nectarines, pitted and quartered; 2 teaspoons of ground coriander; 3 tablespoons or orange marmalade; and 1 tablespoon of snipped fresh thyme.

1) **The glaze:** Combine orange marmalade, thyme, coriander, orange peel, olive oil, and paprika; set aside.

2) On 4 metal skewers, alternate chicken with fruits; grill over medium coals for 6-8 minutes, turning occasionally.

3) Brush chicken kabobs and fruits with glaze; grill for 5 minutes more or until chicken is tender and no longer pink, turning and brushing with glaze occasionally.

4) Season with salt and black pepper; serve. (4 servings)

Chicken Casserole

Calories: 250 per serving

Ingredients:

Rice: 1cup of cooked (in water) long grain rice.

Chicken Ingredients:1 1/2 cups of cubed cooked chicken; 1 can (20 ounces) unsweetened pineapples chunks, drained; 1 jar (12 ounces) apricot preserves or spread able fruit; 1 can (8 ounces) water chestnuts, drained; and 1 can (10.5 ounces) condensed chicken soup, undiluted.

1) Combine all chicken ingredients and bake, uncovered, at 350⁰ F for 30 minutes or until heated through.

2) Serve over cooked rice; season to taste with salt and pepper. (4 servings)

Cheese- Chicken

Calories: 250 per serving

Ingredients:

4 skinless chicken breast halves; 1 pear, cored and cut into 4 thin slices; 4 slices of Swiss cheese; 2 tablespoons of shredded sage; 3 tablespoons of olive oil; and 2 cups of grapefruits.

1) Insert one pear slice, one cheese slice, and 1 teaspoon of the sage on top of the cheese into a pocket made into the chicken breast halves.

2) In a large skillet, cook chicken in hot olive oil until browned, turning once.

3) Pour the grapefruit over the chicken and sprinkle with the remaining sage.

4) Bring to boiling and reduce heat; simmer, covered, for 8-10 minutes or until chicken is tender and no longer pink.

5) Remove chicken from skillet; cover and keep warm.

6) Bring the cooking liquid in skillet into a boil, uncovered, or until liquid is reduced to about 1 cup; serve over chicken. (4 servings)

Sesame Chicken

Calories: 250 per serving

Ingredients:

4 chicken breast halves, cubed; 2 tablespoons olive oil; 1/4 cup soy sauce; 1/4 cup sesame seeds; 1 medium onion, chopped; and 10 ounces of mushroom, sliced, drained.

1) Cook chicken in olive oil until no longer pink in the center.

2) Stir in soy sauce and sesame seeds; cook and stir over medium heat for 5 minutes.

3) Remove chicken with a slotted spoon; set aside and keep warm.

4) In the same skillet, sauté onion and mushrooms until onion is tender; return chicken to pan and heat through.

5) Season to taste with salt and pepper; serve. (4 servings)

STEAK

Flank Steak

Calories: 250 per serving

Ingredients:

Rice: 1 cup of cooked (in water) long grain rice.

Flank Steak ingredients:16 ounces of Flank steak, cut into stripes; 2 tablespoons of olive oil; 2 medium zucchini, julienned; 1 small onion, cut into 1/4 -inch strips; 3 cloves of garlic, minced; 1 cup fresh or frozen peas; 1 cup of sliced mushrooms; 8 ounces of water chestnuts, sliced; and 3 tablespoons of light soy sauce.

1) Cook steak in 1 tablespoon of olive oil until no longer pink in the center; drain and set aside.

2) In the same skillet, sauté onions for 2 minutes; stir in zucchini and garlic for 2 more minutes.

3) Return steak to the skillet and combine soy sauce; bring to boil and cook with stirring until thickened.

4) Serve on rice; season to taste with salt and pepper, if desired. (4 servings)

Salmon Steak

Calories: 250 per serving

Ingredients:

16 ounces of fresh or frozen salmon steaks, cut into 3/4- inch thick; 1 tablespoon of olive oil; 2 tablespoons of grapefruit or orange juice; 3 canned jalapeno pepper, seeded and finely chopped; 1 teaspoon of lemon juice; and 3 tablespoons of Dijon mustard.

1) Thaw salmon steaks, if frozen; rinse and pat dry with paper towels.

2) Glaze: stir the mustard, jalapeno peppers, grapefruit juice, and lemon juice.

3) Lightly brush both sides of salmon steak with the glaze mixture; grill for 6- 9 minutes or until salmon flakes easily when tested with a fork, gently turning and brushing occasionally with the glaze mixture.

4) Season to taste with salt and pepper; serve. (4 servings)

Steak Burritos

Calories: 250 per serving

Ingredients:

16 ounces of flank steak, cut to four portions; 2 envelopes taco seasoning; 1 medium onion, chopped; 1 tablespoon vinegar; 4 flour tortillas (7 inches); 1/2 cup of Monterey Jack cheese; 1 medium tomato, chopped; and1/2 cup fat-free sour cream.

1) Rub the steak portions with taco seasoning; place in a slow cooker coated with nonstick cooking spray.

2) Top the steak with onion, chilies, and vinegar; cover and cook until meat is tender (6- 8 hours).

3) Remove from cooker and shred the steak with two forks; return to cooker and heat through.

4) Spoon about 1/2 cup meat mixture down the center of each tortilla and top with cheese, tomato, and sour cream; fold sides and ends over filling. (4 serving)

Gingered Steak

Calories: 250 per serving

Ingredients:

16 ounces of flank steak; 1 medium onion, chopped; 3 cloves of garlic, minced; 2 tablespoons of olive oil; 1/4 cup of soy sauce; 1/2 teaspoon of ground ginger; and 2 tablespoons of water.

1) In a large re-sealable plastic bag or shallow glass container, combine the soy sauce, water, garlic, olive oil and ginger; mix well.

2) Add steak to the plastic bag mixture and turn to coat; cover, refrigerate for 8 hours or overnight, and drain with discarding marinade.

3)Grill, covered, turning occasionally for 8-10 minutes on each side or until meat reaches desired doneness (for rare, a meat thermometer should read 140^0 F; medium, 160^0 F; well-done,170^0 F).

4) Season to taste with salt and pepper; serve. (4 servings)

Horseradish Steak

Calories: 250 per serving

Ingredients:

16 ounces of beef flank steak, fat trimmed and cut into four portions; 3 tablespoons of Dijon mustard; 5 teaspoons of Worcestershire sauce; 3 tablespoons of lemon juice; 1/2 cup of fat-free dairy sour cream (or fat-free mayonnaise dressing); 2 green onions, finely chopped; and 2 teaspoons of prepared horseradish.

1) **Marinade:** combine 2 tablespoons of the mustard, the lemon juice; and Worcestershire sauce; pour over the steak in a plastic bag and seal the bag.

2) Marinate in the refrigerator for 6 hours to overnight, turning bag occasionally.

3) **The sauce:** Combine remaining mustard, the sour cream, green onion, and horseradish; cover and refrigerate.

4) Remove from refrigerator about 1/2 hour before serving time.

5) Drain steak and discard marinade; grill until desired doneness, turning once halfway through grilling.

6) Serve by thinly slicing steak across the grain; serve with sauce. (4 servings)

Microwave Steak

Calories: 250 per serving

Ingredients:

16 ounces of boneless round steak, cut into 1/2 inch thick cubes and tenderized by pounding with a mallet; 8 ounces of mushroom pieces, drained; 14.5 ounces of diced tomatoes; 4 tablespoons of onion soup mix; and 1/2 teaspoon cayenne pepper.

1) Sprinkle steak with soup mix and mushrooms; separately combine tomatoes and pepper thoroughly.

2) Pour tomato mix over steak; cover and microwave on high for 6-7 minutes or until mixture begins to boil.

3) Turn meat and rotate dish; cover and cook on low for 25 minutes longer or until meat is tender.

4) Season to taste with salt and pepper; serve. (4 servings)

Chili

Chili -Stuffed Peppers

Calories: 250 per serving

Ingredients:

4 medium green peppers, seeded and topped off; 16 ounces of ground beef; 1/2 cup onion, chopped; 15 ounces of chili beans, un-drained; 10 ounces of diced tomatoes and green chilies, un-drained; 1 teaspoon chili powder; 1/2 cup cheddar cheese, shredded; and 1/4 teaspoon of cayenne pepper.

1) Boil green peppers in a large kettle and cook until crisp-tender; drain, rinse, and set aside.

2) Cook beef and onion over medium heat until meat is no longer pink; drain and add beans, tomatoes, chili powder, pepper, and cayenne.

3) Bring to boiling, reduce heat; cover and simmer for 5 minutes.

4) Spoon meat mixture into peppers; cover and bake at 350 F until heated through.

5) Sprinkle with cheese and season to taste; serve. (4 servings)

Cannelloni Chili

Calories: 250 per serving

Ingredients:

16 ounces of skinless chicken breasts, cut into 1/4 -inch cubes; 15 ounces of cannellini (white kidney beans) rinsed and drained; 1 tablespoon of olive oil; 1 medium onion, chopped; 1 cup of low-sodium chicken broth; 4 ounces of chopped green chilies; 1 clove of garlic chopped; 1/2 teaspoon of dried oregano; 1/2 teaspoon of parsley, minced; 1/4 teaspoon of cayenne pepper; and 8 reduced -fat tortilla chips.

1) Sauté chicken and onion in hot oil until juices run clear; drain.

2) Stir in chicken broth, chilies, garlic, oregano, and cayenne; bring to boiling.

3) Reduce heat; simmer, uncovered, for 30 minutes.

4) Stir in beans and cook for 10 minutes longer; Serve over tortilla chips.

Appetizer

Garlic Dip

Calories: 125 per serving

Ingredients:

2 slices of 100% grain bread, toasted; 1/2 cup almonds, toasted; 4 cloves of garlic, finely minced; 2 tablespoon lemon juice; 1 tablespoon of olive oil; 3/4 cup of water; and 2 tablespoons of fresh parsley, chopped.

1) Process (in a food processor or electric blender) the toast bread, almonds, and garlic until finely ground; add the remaining ingredients and process until the mixture is smooth.

2) Scrape the mixture into a bowl, and season to taste with salt and pepper. (4 servings)

Cinnamon Applesauce

Calories: 250 per serving

Ingredients:

6 medium tart apples, peeled and sliced; 1 cup of grapefruit juice; 1 teaspoon of ground cinnamon; 2 cloves of garlic, finely minced; and 1/2 teaspoon of ground allspice.

1) Combine all ingredients, cover, and cook over medium-low heat for 30-40 minutes or until apples are tender.

2) Remove from the heat; mash apples to desired consistency; serve warm or cold. (4 servings)

Middle Eastern Hummus

Calories: 125 per serving

Ingredients:

1/2 cup dried garbanzos (chickpeas); 1/4 cup of water; 1/4 cup of fresh lemon juice; 4 cloves of garlic, finely minced; 1 tablespoon of olive oil; 1/2 cup of sesame Tahini; 1/2 teaspoon of cumin; and 1 teaspoon of baking soda.

1) Soak the garbanzos for 8-10 hours with the baking soda in cold water to cover; bring the beans into a boil, reduce heat, and cook, covered, until soft.

2) Drain, reserving a bit of liquid.

3) Make the Tahini sauce: Blend the Tahini, 1/2 cup cold water, lemon juice, cumin, and garlic.

4) Process garbanzos in a food processor or blender to a rough puree; add the Tahini sauce and process until just mixed.

5) Scrape the mixture into a bowl; stir in the olive oil.

6) Serve with one pita bread, oat bran bead toast, or two carrot sticks. (4 servings)

Chapter 15

Food Preparation

"By the same power that slays you. I too am slain: I too shall be consumed. For the law that delivered you into my hand shall deliver me into a mightier hand. Your blood and my blood is naught but the sap that feeds the tree of heaven."

Khalil Gibran. Poet

I discovered the great benefits of cooking in weekends at the medical school. Actually, I found that cooking is a healing for my anxiety and stress. Preparing food was a cure for my mind and spiritual ills. I found meditation in chopping anions, slicing tomatoes, cleaning chicken of skin, and washing dishes; it's as creating order from chaos. Separating out any extraneous or unusable material is creating order. It's also as a spiritual act by sorting the good parts of vegetable from the bad ones, saving all the best parts for incorporation into my meal and discarding the rest.

Besides creating order from chaos, which was a soothing remedy for a jangled mind's man- barely above his teen years in medical school, food preparation constituted a kind of magic that has great applications in other areas of life. It's fascinating to create a nice dish from raw ingredients with a virtual picture or verbal description- it includes imagined aromas and flavors. It's a thrilling to add ingredients by handfuls, smatterings and smidgeons rather than in measured amounts. It's a challenge to create delicious dishes with spices and herbs by tasting rather than by referring to recipes. Actually, cooking is a real magic that translates a mere vision into a delicious reality. I need to emphasize that I do not mean to downplay the fact that cooking requires effort and time when I describe the rewards and pleasure of cooking. It's much easier to enjoy cooking when Mom is an award-winning in cooking in her teens as mine; genetic! Or imprinting! Or both! My cooking experience is not always rosy- especially cooking fires from unattended cooking.

159

In this section, I will discuss four major topics.

1) Wild Game Meats,

2) Grading of Meat in America,

3) Food-Transmitted Diseases, and

4) Food Storage and Cooking.

Wild Game Meats

Hunting Field Necessities: A functional rifle and enough shells, sharp hunting knife, small hatchet, whetstone or steel, 12 -18 feet of light rope, plastic bags, lots of paper towels, binoculars, canteen of fresh water, compass, map, matches, and most of all a license for hunting in public land. Moreover, cheesecloth and red hot pepper are needed to repel flies in hot weathers; long boots and socks are needed to protect from deer ticks, and orange-colored apparel and hat are needed to warn others from shooting you.

Bleeding the Animal

Bleed, dress and cool the carcass promptly. Internal bleeding into the chest cavity may be enough for animals shot in the ribs. Although other shots require no other additional bleeding, severing the large blood vessel leading to the heart improves bleeding and food appearance.

Field Dressing: As soon the animal is dead, 1) remove intestines, liver, heart. 2) Keep the carcass clean and use clean utensils during dressing. 3) Cool the carcass quickly, during processing and transport. 4) Wear gloves to prevent disease (Prion-caused diseases) transmission. 5) Wash hands and knife frequently to prevent meat contamination during field dressing. 6) Cut the animal and do not save organ meat (brain and liver) because they are cholesterol-rich organs.7) and refrigerate the meat promptly.

Aging Meat: Hold the meat or carcass at 34 to 37^0 F for 7 to 14 days to allow the enzymes in the meat to break down some of the complex proteins in the carcass. Aged meat is often more tender and flavorful. Aging is not recommended for young animals and fat thin-covered animals because they may dry out during aging and become more susceptible to deterioration through microbial growth. Do not remove hide or trim fat from game meat before aging because the hide and fat protect against dehydration. If meat will be ground into sausage, aging is not necessary.

Cold Shortening: When the internal muscle temperature drops to 32^0 F within hours of the kill, such conditions cause meat toughness. Frozen carcasses should be thawed and aged at 34^0 F for 14 days.

Marinades: Marinades can tenderize, enhance or disguise game flavors to fit your preference. Cover meat with one of the following marinades and allow standing in the refrigerator at least 24 hours and then broil, roast or braise.

1) 2 cups vinegar and 2 cups of water

2) French dressing and tomato sauce

3) Fruit juice (lemon or pineapple)

4) 1.4 cup vinegar, 1/2 cup canola oil, 1/2 teaspoon red pepper, 1/2 teaspoon garlic

5) 2 tablespoons of vinegar, 1 1/2 teaspoon ground ginger, 2 tablespoons of garlic, 1/2 cup of soy sauce, and 3/4 cup of olive oil.

Nutrient Content of wild game: All wild game meats have about 150 calories/ 100 grams of meat (3 1/2 ounces) and 80 milligrams of cholesterol. However, there are some exceptions.

The following animals are high in cholesterol (mg/ 100 gram of meat)

Pig (wild Boar) - 109 mg, widgeon -131 mg, rabbit (Jack) - 131 mg, goose (Sage) - 101 mg, goose (Sow) - 141 mg, duck (Mallard) - 140 mg, deer (whitetail) - 116 mg, crane (Sand hill) - 123 mg, and antelope- 112 mg.

Composition of fat in game meat

Large-Size Animals

	SFA (%)	MUSFA (%)	PUNSFA (%)
Buffalo	43	45	12
Elk	48	27	25
Moose	37	24	39
Caribou	47	36	17

Medium -Size Animals

	SFA (%)	MUSFA (%)	PUNSFA (%)
Antelope	41	27	32
Pig (Boar)	36	47	17
Deer (Mule)	48	32	20
Deer (Whitetail)	46	30	24

Small-Size Animals

	SFA (%)	MUSFA (%)	PUSFA (%)
Squirrel	15	47	38
Rabbit	39	36	25

SFA, Saturated fatty acids; MUSFA, monounsaturated fatty acids; and PUSFA, polyunsaturated fatty acids

Grading of Meat in America

After the meat and poultry are inspected for wholesomeness, producers and processors may request to have the products graded for quality by a federal grader. Grading for quality requires evaluation for tenderness, juiciness, and flavor of meat; for poultry, the normal shape that is fully fleshed and meaty and free of defects.

USDA Grades for Meat and Poultry

Beef

Beef is graded as whole carcasses in two ways:

*Quality grades- for tenderness, juiciness, and flavor. Quality grades are based on the amount of marbling (flecks of fat within the lean), color, and maturity; and

*Yield grades- for the amount of usable lean meat on the carcass.

Quality grades:

*Prime grade- is produced from young, well-fed beef cattle with abundant marbling. Generally sold to hotels and restaurants; prime roasts and steaks are excellent for dry-heat cooking (i.e. roasting, broiling and grilling).

*Choice grade- is high quality with less marbling. Choice roasts and steaks from the lion and rib will be very tender, juicy and flavorful. Choice grades are good for dry -heat (145^0 F (medium rare); 160^0 F (medium); and 170^0 F (well done).

*Select grade- is very uniform in quality and normally leaner than the higher grades. It is very tender, but has less marbling and lacks juiciness and flavor.

Yield grades: range from 1 to 5 and indicate the amount of usable meat from a carcass. Yield 1 is the highest and denotes the greatest ratio of lean to fat; yield 5 is the lowest yield ratio. Yield grade is the most useful when purchasing a side or carcass of beef for the freezer.

Tender Cuts	Tough Cuts
Tenderloin steak	Bottom round steak
Top lion steak	Top round roast
Top blade steak	Round tip steak
Rib roast	Chick tender steak
Rib steak	Rump steak
Cold roast	Bottom round steak

Top sirloin steak　　　Top round steak

Rib eye steak　　　　Eye of round roast

Poultry

USDA grades poultry as A, B and C.

*Grade A- is the highest quality and the only grade that is likely to be seen at the retail level. This grade indicates that the products are virtually free from defects such as bruises, discolorations, and feathers. Bone-in products have no broken bones. For whole birds and parts with the skin on, there are no tears in the skin or exposed flesh that could dry out during cooking, and there is a good covering of fat under the skin. Moreover, whole birds and parts will be fully fleshed and meaty.

The grade shield for poultry may be found on the following chilled or frozen ready-to-cook poultry products: whole carcasses and products, as well as roasts, tenderloins, and other boneless and/ or skinless poultry products that are being marketed. There are no grade standards for necks, wing tips, tails, giblets, or ground poultry.

*Grades B and C- is usually used in further- processed products where the poultry meat is cut up, chopped, or ground. If sold in retail, they are usually not grade identified. Should you have any further questions, contact meat and poultry hotline?

1-888-674-6854 -Toll free or 1-800-256-7072 (TDD/TTY) or

Email: mphotline.fsis@USDA.gov

Factors That Affect Meat Tenderness

Minor factors

a) Genetics: Brahman breed lacks meat tenderness and Piedmonts pass on very good tenderness traits when cross bred to Angus and Hereford, but the same crosses with the Nellore breed as a sire were found to be relatively tough. In general only 30% of the tenderness of meat can be ascribed to all forms of genetic factors.

b) Pasture effect: pasture influences the pH of the meat; for example, sheep meat that is very high or very low in pH is tender, but a high- pH- sheep- meat is dark and often has a 'rubbery' texture. Low- pH meat, also tender, does not have this undesirable texture.

Major factors

a) Stress: Stress prior slaughter affects meat tenderness and pH level. Stressed animals have a pH around 5.5 (acidic) after 24 hours of death because all sugars have been converted.

B) Electrical stunning- Electrical stunning immediately prior to slaughter improves tenderness, mainly through mechanically fracturing some of the giant, intermediate and shorter muscle fibers of meat.

c) Aging: Very rapid chilling immediately after slaughter causes toughness. Aging for 7 to 14 days at 35- 40⁰ F after kill improves tenderness.

d) Age: Young animals are much tender because the protein breaking down enzyme system decreases as the animal gets older and collagen increases.

e) Marinating: papaya fruits, which contain a protein breaking down enzyme called " papain' and kiwi fruit have similar proteolysis enzymes have a tenderness effect on surface. Crude ginger extract at 0.5 to 1.0 5 levels in the marinating improves meat tenderness by 20-30% in the absence of 2% salt and by 35-45% in the presence of 2% salt.

f) Vitamin D: Vitamin injection or fed with vitamin D (7.5 million IU* of vitamin D3) for 7 days before slaughter improves meat tenderness.

g) Calcium: Injection of calcium chloride before slaughter into the carcass through veins and arteries improves meat tenderness.

h) Hydro dyne: placing a carcass in water and then setting off a controlled explosion in the water instantly tenderizes the carcass.

*IU, International unit.

Food Storage and Cooking

Thiamin (vitamin B_1) is used by the body to keep nerves in healthy conditions; it stimulates a good appetite. Beriberi, a disease characterized by weakness and inflamed nerves, was common in Orientals because of their polished rice diet. Polishing rice removes the husks containing thiamin. Thiamin is found in whole grain, pork, yeast, and fresh green vegetables.

Thiamin is destroyed by as much as 22% boiled in some vegetables in water and additional amounts up to 15% dissolved in the cooking water. When cooking water is discarded total thiamin losses in vegetables may account to approximately 20 to 35%. Addition of a small amount of sodium bicarbonate markedly increased the destruction of thiamin content of boiled navy beans.

Roasting causes a loss of 43% of the thiamin in pork loin, nearly three times as much loss as braising.

Double boiler cooking of whole grain cereals did not destroy thiamin; baking bread caused about 15% loss of thiamin.

Chapter 16

Drinking Water

"I have never seen a hearse with a luggage rack."

Randy Travis, Country singer

Environmental Protection Agency (EPA) regulates pollutants treated as carcinogens in the range of 10^{-6} to 10^{-4} (or 1 in 10,000) to protect average exposed individuals. Some people are vulnerable to water contaminants than the general public. Immune-compromised persons such as persons under chemotherapy for cancer, persons who have under-gone organ transplants, people with HIV/AIDS or other immune system disorders, some elderly and infants vulnerable to pollutants' effects.

Drinking water, including bottled water, may reasonably expect to contain at least small amounts of some contaminants. Community (public) water systems are required to disclose the detection of these contaminants; however, bottled water companies are not required regularly to comply with this regulation!

Sources of Public Water Contaminations

Soil Runoff: Causes turbidity. Turbidity in excess of 5 NTU is just noticeable to the average person.

Plumbing Systems: Copper and lead are the major contaminants from plumbing systems. Use stainless pipes or cPVC pipes not copper pipes in plumbing.

Fertilizers: Fluoride (1- 1.99 ppm), nitrate (safe levels are 10 parts per million- ppm), and nitrite (safe levels not to exceed 1 ppm) are the major contaminants of fertilizers. Nitrates and nitrites are produced from many industries, such as fertilizer plants, metal ores, explosives, paper mills, pulp mills, canned foods and phosphate fertilizers.

Water Treatment: Fluoride, chlorine, halo acetic acids, trihalomethanes, and sodium.

Microorganisms: Untreated drinking water may contain:

Shigella dysenteria, Vibrio cholerae, Yersinia enterocolitica, Aeromonas hydrophilis, Campylobacter jejuni, Eschererchia coli, Salmonella typhi, Legionella pnuemophilia, Kleibsiella terigena, Poliovirus type 1, Hepatitis A virus, *Saccharomyces cerevisiae,* Rotavirus SA-11, *and Bacillus substillis.* ***Cooking food at 165F or above kills all organisms, including Salmonella.***

Learn more about your drinking water by contacting:

1) EPAs Safe Drinking Water Hotline: 800- 424-4791

2) Chemicals in you area: Community Right-to- Know Hotline 800-424-9346

Fluoride Toxicity

The Food and Nutrition Board recommends that public water supplies be fluoridated when natural fluoride levels are below 0.7 mg per liter. The accepted concentration of fluoride in drinking water is between 1 to 1.99 ppm; concentration of fluoride above 2 ppm is a health risk. Many municipal water supplies are treated with alum (aluminum sulfate) and fluoride. When these two chemicals combine, they form aluminum fluoride that is poorly secreted in the urine. It is poisonous to the kidneys; aluminum salts in the brain lead to Alzheimer's disease. Fluoride intake of 20-40 mg/day can inhibit phosphates (enzyme) that is required for calcium utilization.

Chapter 17

Cop-outs

"Let us free of government hold; it's our right," said John Doe at GW. The professor answered, "Everyone's right is guaranteed as long as three conditions are met:1) his or her rights do not infringe on others' rights, 2) others have no invested interests on it and 3) do not cause burden on or harm o to others. The professor proceeded with the following questionnaires to determine whether others have the right to limit your freedom or not:

1) Since your health insurance is either paid by your employer as tax-deductable business expenses or by subsidy from the federal or state governments which is tax-payers' money, should the government should limit such deductions by your employer? (Only 17% of Americans own a profitable business.)

2) Since we have a federal law for hospitals not to deny you healthcare regardless whether you have health insurance or not and the federal or state government end up paying your healthcare costs, if indigent, should the federal or state government require you to have healthcare insurance? (95% of Americans' health insurance is subsidized by tax-payers' money; your own congressman and US senator's health insurance premiums are 75% subsidized by tax-payers' money. All non-profit, tax-exempt organizations (worship, educational or political receive government grants and tax-exempt donations.)

3) Since intoxicated and stoned drivers have higher chances of vehicle fatal accidents, should the government make it illegal to drive while intoxicated or stoned? (Obese, intoxicated and stoned drivers have four times as much as non-obese, non-intoxicated or non-stoned drivers' accidents.)

4) Since the country has an interest on citizens with high educational skills to meet the country's security interests, should the government set educational standards for its students in k-12? (During the Iraq War, the Pentagon initiated Stop Gap for lack of physically and educationally fit volunteers to the military.)

5) Since we share air, water and roads, should the government set standards to curb pollution and wear and tear on our highways and waterways?

Constitutionally, you have the rights to practice speech, religion, assembly because all those freedoms cost nothing to others. Also you have the right to carry firearms to stop tyrannical government, and the right to counsel, if indigent, to assure justice to others. John Doe shouted angrily, "I am only free on the moon if I can get there or live in a cave alone without any needs or share with others."

Weight-loss cop- out methods: a) Prescription drugs

b) Plastic Surgery   c) Bariatric Surgery

Prescription Drugs

I need to emphasize that life style changes or drugs alone will usually get you 7 percent loss of your total weight without difficulty. However, life changes combined with drugs will get you 14 percent loss of your total weight. Never forget the side effects of prescription drugs for weight loss; their benefits must outweigh their side effects and should not be used for cosmetic weight loss. These drugs are approved for BMI above 30 or 27 with obesity related conditions like high blood pressure and diabetes.

One of the newest drugs of **appetite control** is cannabinoid blockers; it prevents cannabinoid receptors from making you hungry. Cannobinoid receptors are the same receptors activated when you smoke marijuana (*Cannabis sativa*).This drug blocks CCK and leptin and reduces craving. Cannabinoid receptors are also found in your liver, belly fat and muscle. Their blockage results in less fat in blood (triglycerides), less risk of diabetes, and more HDL cholesterol. The downside of this drug is that you may revert to your old habit of foraging everything when you come off them.

Caffeine and nicotine as **appetite suppressants**, they increase nor-epinephrine (the fight-or-flight phyto-chemical), suppressing appetite, and speeding hear rate. You need to weigh the risk of smoking cigarettes against your desire to lose weight. Nicotine patches and gums with two cups of coffee daily are good waist management cocktail. Sibutramine (Meridia) suppresses appetite by acting like serotonin, so you do not experience the sudden surge and decrease in brain chemicals that lead to hedonistic eating. Zelnorm (tegaserod) is another drug that stimulates serotonin; which makes you feel good and consequently eat less.

Gastric -emptying drugs: CCK and chemical- likes injection or inhalation can cause feeling of fullness by slowing gastric-emptying and may help increase satiety levels.

Blocking digestion of fat drugs: Xenical (Orlistat) works by inhibiting the enzyme lipase, which is responsible for breaking down dietary fat for bile action and absorption. When fat is not broken down, the body cannot absorb it, so you take in fewer calories. The downside of Xenical is that you absorb less of the fat-soluble vitamins A, D, and E from your food. Another side is more frequent stools and more gas. Further, addiction is another consideration.

Blocking digestion of carbohydrates drugs: Acarbose (Precose) inhibits an enzyme in metabolism of carbohydrates; therefore, no breakdown of carbohydrates and no absorption by your body. The down sides are diarrhea and fermentation of sugars, resulting in more gas.

Activating CCK drugs: Zantac (over the counter drug) is an acid - relieving drug and it may work by activating CCK, so that you feel full. Some studies have shown that Cimetidine (the prescription acid relief form of Zantac (Vanitidine), in a dose of 400 milligrams three times a day, may decrease waist size by 5 percent.

Plastic Surgery

Surgery	Number of patients/ year	Cost in US dollars
Liposuction	480,000	2,000 per area
Breast Augmentation	320,000	5,000- 8,000
Eyelid Surgery	300,000	4,000- 5,500
Rhinoplasty	170,000	5,000- 6,000
Face-lift	160,000	7,000 - 9,000

In addition to the economic burden that is not usually covered by health insurance, the surgery is not going to correct your already stretched body. Moreover, some of these surgeries, liposuction, would not help you lose a significant weight.

Bariatric Surgery

This surgery is for somebody whose body mass index is 35 or higher, with diabetes and hypertension. The success of surgery is defined by continuous weight loss of 50% of your excess weight. By this definition, surgery has a success rate of more than 90% at one year, with an average over five years between 55- 70 %. These surgeries are irreversible and need a commitment to taking vitamin B_{12}; drinking lots of water; no or little alcohol, caffeine, soda, and acidic foods; and not drinking during meals to stay healthy for the rest of your life.

a) Gastric Banding: Restrictive

A belt - like band is tightened up high around the stomach. This band constricts the stomach and leaves a very small pouch at the top of the stomach for food storage as it enters from the esophagus. Basically, this band limits your access to food by limiting your intake. It is reversible.

b) Duodenal Switch

In this procedure, the intestines are cut and reattached, to quicken the time for food passage through the intestine and not all the nutrients are fully absorbed; up to 80% of the intestine is cut. There is a possibility of leakage in your body and the need for nutrient supplementation.

c) Gastric Pacing

A gastric pacemaker is placed on the stomach near the Vagus nerve. This pacemaker sends signals to the brain that you are full by mimicking the actions of CCK. It is less invasive procedure without any cuts at all.

Chapter 18

Dietary Therapy

Let food be your medicine and medicine be your food."   Hippocrates

1) Digestive System Problems

a) Anemia

1) Increase intake of vitamin C (in kiwi and citrus fruits); and 2) Increase intake of red meat and dried beans, dried fruits, molasses and cocoa.

b) Diarrhea

1) Avoid milk and milk products, caffeine and sugar foods until problems subside.

c) Diverticulitis

1) Increase dietary fiber especially whole wheat grains; 2) drink plenty of water (4- 6 cups daily); and 3) Avoid caffeine.

D) Constipation

1) Drink plenty of water (4- 6 cups of water daily); and 2) Increase intake of high -fiber foods, such as vegetables, fruits, and whole-grain bread.

E) Scurvy: Spongy gums, loosened teeth, and bleeding under skin.

Eat lots of vitamin C- rich foods such as kiwi and citrus fruits.

f) Irritable Bowel Syndrome

1) Eliminate milk and milk products, all caffeine sources, and sweeteners; and 2) Increase dietary fiber by eating more whole-grain breads, fruits and vegetables.

g) Liver Problems

1) Decrease protein and fat intake to 20 - 30% or less of daily calorie intake; and 2) Avoid alcohol and caffeine.

h) Ulcer (peptic Ulcer)

1) Avoid milk, milk products, caffeine, and alcohol; 2) Eat smaller and more frequent meals; and 3) Eat some hot red pepper and plenty of fruit and vegetables.

I) Heartburn: Acid reflux disease

1) Chew gum to neutralize the acidity of the stomach, avoid caffeine, and drink orange juice or apple juice; 2) Eat fresh fruits and vegetables; 3) Avoid taking Aspirin in empty stomach; 4) Drink a 1/2 cup of warm water before and after taking Aspirin; and 5) Eat food in small quantity and do not lie down right after meal.

j) Hemorrhoids (piles)

Relieve constipation and drink plenty of water. Exercise regularly.

K) Alcohol intoxication (alcohol level over 0.02)

The longer the alcohol remains in the stomach, the more slowly the blood alcohol level rises. Blood alcohol level will rise more slowly when fat-rich foods, such as meat, nuts, or fish are consumed together with alcohol- containing drinks. Female often experience higher blood alcohol levels and therefore become drunk faster than males of comparable size because females have a smaller total body fluid volume and the alcohol dehydrogenase (enzyme that breaks down alcohol) is up to 60% lower in females and Asian males than in other males.

L) Jaundice: A yellowish coloration of the sclera of the eyes and skin.

1) Liver in newborns functions poorly for the first week or so, many babies experience neonatal jaundice that disappears as the liver matures. Usually, jaundice is treated by exposing the infant to blue light. In adults, jaundice is caused by hepatitis infection or cirrhosis; and 2) Avoid alcohol intake and take

174

hepatitis B vaccine early in life. Our neighbor died at young age from hepatitis B because he refused at ten years old to go with his mother to their family doctor for a Hepatitis B vaccine. Avoidance is better than treatment: follow your doctor's advice to save your life and save scarce healthcare dollars on complicated health problems that you should have taken care of earlier in life.

M) Gallbladder Problems

1) Reduce animal protein; 2) Eat calcium-rich foods such as shellfish and green leafy vegetables; 3)Reduce dietary cholesterol to no more than 300 milligrams a day; cholesterol - rich foods are egg yolk, brain, liver, cow's milk (5.5% fat) and bison's (buffalo) milk (7.5 % fat); and 4) Cut down on fat -rich foods.

2) Skeleton System Problems

A) Athlete's foot: a parasitic fungus disease.

1) Chlorinated foot baths leading to swimming pools helps to retard the spread of the fungus; 2) Dry toes thoroughly with the aid of a foot powder; 3) Decrease sugar intake and eat lots of garlic (preferably fresh or cooked lightly); and 4) Sprinkle some oregano in your food every day. Oregano has antiseptic power and is indefinitely more potent than commercial phenol in its microbial killing power. Phenol is carcinogen too.

B) Gout: a joint inflammation.

1) Eliminate caffeine and alcohol; and 2) Reduce animal protein intake to 20% of the daily calorie intake.

c) Osteoporosis

1) Replace dietary animal protein with plant protein (nuts, seeds, soy, and vegetables); 2) Eat lots of broccoli and green leafy vegetables that are rich in calcium, especially spinach; and 3) Sunlight exposure of 15- 20 minutes daily helps with weight - bearing exercise (walking). Sunlight provides vitamin D, which

is essential in metabolism of calcium. Further note: Vitamin D supplement pills are not as effective as rich-calcium nutrients or exposure to sunlight because nutritional supplements pill contains both active and non-active forms of vitamin D.

d) Multiple Sclerosis: A progressive destruction of myelin sheaths of the neurons. It is a disabling disease that affects 2.6 million people worldwide.

1) Eat lots of vitamin C- rich foods, such as kiwi, red seeded - grapes, and citrus fruits; and 2) Cook with canola and olive oils.

E) Rheumatoid Arthritis: an autoimmune disease in which the immune system of the body attacks its own tissues.

1) Eat lots of fish and two teaspoons of cold-pressed flax seed daily; 2) Cook with canola and olive oils; 3) Walk daily for a 1/2 hour and do stretch exercise for 5- 10 minutes after walking; and 4) sprinkle a 1/8 teaspoon of turmeric in your food every day.

F) Lyme disease

It is caused by a spiral-shaped bacterium (*Borrelia burgdorferi*) transmitted to humans mainly by deer ticks (*Ixodes dammini*) that are so small and most often their bites go unnoticed. Avoid ticks in hunting areas (timber) and cook thoroughly game meat.

3) Others

A) Cancer

1) Eat lots of broccoli, blueberry, apple, and carrots for antioxidant agents; 2) Avoid drinking coffee; 3) Eat lots of mushrooms, especially *Cordyceps sinesis*, *Ganoderma lucidum* (Reishi), *Agaricus spp*, and *Coriolus versicolor*; 4) Drink red wine (for Resveratrol); 5) Eat lots of garlic, grain cereals, chicken, and sea foods for (selenium); 6) Eat dark chocolate with at least 70% cocoa (antioxidant), and goji berries; 7) Walk for a 1/2 hour daily in sunlight for vitamin D; 8) drink green or black tea for epigallocatechin (EGCG); 9) avoid eating stale grains such as corn, wheat, barley, sorghum, and nuts because they are commonly contaminated with the cancer-causing fungal poisons (aflatoxin); 10) Eat live yogurt with the transient beneficial

bacteria; 11) Avoid highly chlorinated water- excess fluoride in treated drinking water is toxic as well as carcinogen; 12) Avoid dental amalgam mercury- fillings because mercury is a potent carcinogen; 13) Avoid mercury-containing vaccines- not true that vaccination cause cancer or dyslexia; we are not in a banana republic; 14) Stay away from tanning salons and long exposure to sunlight between 10 A.M and 4 P.M. because of carcinogenic effect of ultraviolet lights, which are intense between 10 A.M and 4 P.M. in the northern hemisphere (0N – 90 N)- mainland America (22N to 45N) is in the northern hemisphere because it lies North of the equator; 15) treat hiatus hernia because it leads to poor digestion and excess toxicity; 16) Use organically grown produce whenever possible because they are grown without herbicides; 17) Avoid polyunsaturated fatty acids and *trans* fatty acids; 18) Use only hormone-free, organically produced meat, poultry, and dairy products; 19) reduce animal fat; and 20) Finally, have faith in God's mercy.

b) Cholesterol Problems

1) Reduce ratio of saturated and polyunsaturated fats to monosaturated fats and omega -3 fatty acids (canola oils, olive oils, safflower oils, and fish); 2) Soy products, garlic and soluble fiber all have shown to lower LDL cholesterol levels. Garlic intake reduces LDL cholesterol levels by up to 9% and produces a small rise in HDL cholesterol levels; one medium -size garlic clove daily is sufficient. Garlic has no known side effects except for the presence of odor in some individuals; 3) Minimize intake of refined, processed foods (cookies and pies) and polyunsaturated fats (such as corn oil, soybean oil, and much margarine); 4) Increase consumption of soluble-fiber, such as whole-grain breads and oat bran. Studies have shown one daily serving of oat bran or oatmeal decreases total cholesterol by up to 3 %; 5) Eat lots of garlic (preferably fresh or cooked lightly), red pepper (Chile), and cooked shiitake mushrooms frequently; 6) Drink green or black tea regularly; 7) Eat lots of blueberries, apples, kiwis, and citrus fruits; 8) Monounsaturated fats (e.g., hazelnuts, almonds, pecans, cashews, walnuts and macadamia nuts) are preferable to nut- containing polyunsaturated fats,

such as peanuts and pine nuts; 9) Stay away from eating cholesterol-rich food (e.g., egg yolk, brain, liver, bison milk - 7.5% fats, cow milk -5.5% fats); 10) Walk daily for a 1/2 hour and do stretch exercise for 5-10 minutes after walking; 11) Garlic, red wine, monounsaturated fats, and fruits and vegetables are associated with decreased oxidation of LDL cholesterol; and 12 Take niacin (vitamin B) 4 times a day; niacin is a natural vitamin to increase HDL. Actually, it is the same niacin prescribed to alleviate cholesterol problems. Niacin (nicotinamide) is found in yeast, meats, fish, whole-grain products, peas, beans, and nuts.

c) Bladder Problems

1) Avoid caffeine in coffee, tea, and cola sodas, which inhibit sodium reabsorption; 2) avoid alcohol in beer, wine, and mixed drinks, which inhibit secretion of ADH (hormone) because they increase the rate of urine flow; and 3) Avoid red and black pepper and decrease sugar in all forms.

D) Bad Breath

1) Eat at least 3--4 hours before bedtime to allow food digestion; 2) Avoid sweet foods at dinner; 3) Chew gum regularly because it helps to clean teeth mechanically and through secretion of saliva; 4) Eat yogurt or take bifidus and acidophilus to add beneficial bacteria and improve digestion; 5) Take a tablespoon of apple cider vinegar before each meal to increase hydrochloric acid in the stomach and improve digestion; 6) Increase intake of high- fiber diets such as whole-grain and fruits and vegetables to optimize digestion; 7) Drink 6-8 glasses of water daily; 8) Increase your intake of vitamin B_6 intake in your diet; 9) Gargle with water to clean out bacteria, mucus and food particles on your tonsils or the back of your throat; and 10) Check with your dentist, if the problems persist.

E) Body Odor

1) Avoid caffeine and decrease animal protein in diet

F) Hypertension

1) Increase intake of fruits and vegetables; 2) Eat lots of garlic-2-3 cloves a day- preferably fresh or lightly cooked; 3) Avoid salty and processed foods; 4) Avoid high -glycemic carbohydrate foods; 5) Avoid cholesterol-rich foods, such as egg yolk, brain, liver and whole milk; and 6) Walk daily for a 1/2 hour and do stretch exercise for 5-10 minutes after walking.

g) Thyroid Problems:

1) Eat sea foods to provide iodine deficiency; 2) Use iodized salt; and 3) Limit intake of soybeans since it can interfere with thyroid function.

h) Prostate Problems

1) Follow all recommendations under cancer prevention; 2) Avoid caffeine sources (coffee and sodas), alcohol, and black and red pepper; 3) Eat whole-grain breads, nuts, and pumpkin seeds; 4) Eat plenty of fresh fruits and vegetables; 5) Add turmeric into your foods (1/8 teaspoon) daily; 6) Drink lots of green tea; 7) Exercise regularly for a 1/2 hour and 5-10 minutes of stretch exercise after walking; 8) Cut down on all processed foods and saturated fats; 9) The bark of the tree (*Pygeum africanum*) from the mountains of southern Africa has been found to relieve prostate enlargement. Saw palmetto and *Pygeum africanum* mix is an excellent relief for prostate enlargement by 50% decrease in urination during the night hours, 26% increase in maximum urinary flow, 45% reduction in residual urine, 62% reduction in painful urination, and 53% reduction in post urination dripping; 10) Lycopene (in Tomatoes)- a Harvard study found that eating tomato products twice a week had a 21% to 34% reduced risk of prostate cancer; and 11) Selenium in mushrooms, seafood and garlic is another powerful agent against prostate enlargement.

I) Kidney Problems

1) Decrease protein intake to maximum of 20% of total daily calorie intake; 2) Replace animal protein in diet with plant proteins such as nuts, seeds, and beans; 3) Limit dietary fat to

25% of daily caloric intake; 4) Drink 4-6 cups of water daily; and 5) Exercise daily for a 1/2 hour of walking followed by a 5-10 minutes of stretch exercise.

J) Menopause (usually between 45- 55 of age in women)

1) Increase intake of calcium -rich foods such as leafy green vegetables, reduced fat, fortified milk, and seafoods; 2) Black cohosh root (80 milligrams) reduces LH levels and improves hot flashes. No scientific studies are available for the effect of black cohosh's use beyond 6 months; and 3) Exercise daily for a 1/2 hour of walking and 5-10 minutes of stretch exercise after walking.

K) Inflammatory Bowel diseases (Colitis and Crohn's disease)

1) Eliminate milk and milk products; 2) Avoid raw vegetables and fruits; 3) Avoid sweeteners with sorbitol or xylitol; 4) Eliminate all caffeine sources, such as coffee, tea, and cola sodas; 5) Exercise regularly for a 1/2 hour of walking and 5-10 minutes of stretch exercise after walking; and 6) Add turmeric (1/8 teaspoon) into your meals.

L) Fibromyalgia

1) Add ginger, mushrooms, and turmeric regularly to food dishes; 2) Eat lots of fruits and vegetables, especially kiwi, citrus fruits, and red- seeded grapes; and 3) Increase intake of omega-3 fatty acids (canola oil, olive oil and fish).

M) Hypoglycemia

1) Avoid high-glycemic -index carbohydrate foods; 2) Avoid saturated fats; 3) Exercise regularly for a 1/2 hour of walking and 5-10 minutes of stretch exercise after walking; and 4) Include low-glycemic- index foods at every meal until the problem subsides.

N) Herbal Remedies of Bad Breath

Chewing anise, cardamom, dill or fennel seeds masks the odor and licorice-flavored seed kills the bacteria that cause mouth odor. Chewing filberts (hazelnuts), mint, parsley, basil, thyme and wintergreen mitigates bad breath. Finally, sucking lemon or cinnamon bark relieves bad breath.

O. Ocular Neuropathy (inflammation of the optic nerve)

Ocular neuropathy has many causes, such as blockage drainage of Cerebral Spinal Fluid (CSF) and Nocturnal hypotension. The latter is characterized pathologically by 26% decrease in systolic blood pressure and 33% decrease in diastolic blood pressure or 60 mmHg or less of arterial blood pressure (systolic) at night. Nocturnal hypotension usually results in vision problems, and it is the result of many physiological and microbial imbalances. Nocturnal hypotension has many causes: Food allergy, food toxicity, prescription- drug side effects, or vector-borne diseases.

a) **Food Allergy**

Vegetable oil, zucchini, pumpkin, pea, and fennel cause allergic reactions that result in nocturnal hypotension.

b) **Food Poisoning**

Apple-seed and sassafras oil and niacin are the main food poisons that cause nocturnal hypotension.

c) **Vector-Borne Diseases**

Malaria (mosquito- borne disease)

d) **Prescription-drug side effects**

Beta blockers and other oral hypertensive therapeutic drugs, especially intensive hypertensive therapy at evening or at bedtime

e) **Dietary life style**

High salty (high sodium) diets and dehydration (lack of intake of adequate water daily- 4-6 cups intake of water daily is needed) and poor diet.

f) **Microbial infections**

Streptococcus and *Staphylococcus* infections

Treatment of Nocturnal Hypotension

1) Increase potassium intake (eat lots of banana) and decrease intake of salty (high sodium) intake. Table salt is sodium chloride.

2) Take a baby Aspirin daily (300 mg) to suppress prostaglandins.

3) Exercise daily (light walk for 30 minutes) to regulate blood pressure and increase myocardial contraction or heart rate.

4) Eat protein and increase intake of vitamin C, fresh fruits, and vitamin B complex- rich foods.

5) Decrease intake of fructose (grape seeds, corn syrup, most soft drinks, and beer are rich in fructose).

6) Stay warm to increase vasodilatation- cold weather increases blood pressure because of vasoconstriction, especially among senior citizens (60 years and older).

7) Increase oxygen intake by decreasing snoring during sleep. Snoring is caused by blockage of the airway by the soft palate tissue. Forwarding of the jaw during sleep decreases soft palate tissue blockage. Raise the pillow (two pillows usually suffice) or just breath from your nose not from mouth (closed mouth during sleeping eliminates snoring and sleep apnea); Listerine gargle before bedtime helps to dry the soft palate and prevent blockage; devices to hold the jaw forward and surgical correction of soft palate tissue are just a few to prevent snoring and therefore decrease nocturnal hypotension.

8) Lowering the head position in comparison to the axis of the body helps to raise nocturnal blood pressure (lower extremities are higher than head − angle of 70 degrees). Gravity pulls blood flow down into the axial and head areas.

Chapter 19

Frequently Asked Questions

"It is only the warlike power of civilized people that can give peace to the world."
                                                                    Theodore Roosevelt

Did you know?

* The average person produces between 100- 150 million sperms in one ejaculate of semen.

* The semen's alkalinity (pH) is 7.2 to 7.7 and semen liquefaction of more than two hours indicates inflammation of sex glands.

Q. What is so unique about the Koreans' and Japanese's diets to make them the slimmest people on earth?

A. They eat lots of fish, fresh fruits, and vegetables and less of the processed food we eat every day. They exercise voluntary or involuntary (working hard) and they have no stressful life like ours. Our Western diet is full of the mostly inflammatory ingredients such as omega- 6 fatty acids and lacks the anti-inflammatory ingredients such as omega 3 fatty acids. We consume forty times omega -6 fatty acids as much as omega-3 fatty acids. The optimum ratio of omega -6 to omega-3 is 4: 1.This imbalance makes our bodies too inflamed. What is the solution? More fish, flaxseed, olive oil, and canola oil in our western diet. Omega -3 fatty acids are also found in fortified eggs, pumpkin, soybean, and cold-water fish as mackerel, sardines, salmon, and tuna.

Q. I am on diabetes medications; is it possible to stay away from diabetes medications if I eat right?

A. 90% of diabetes is caused by type II (over 40 of age) as a result of insulin level's imbalance. Eat proteins and fats that come from vegetables and fruits like avocado, olive oil, nuts, beans, kiwi, red- seeded grapes, grapefruit and soy; avoid processed foods such as cookies and pies; and eat whole grain breads. Try to make your meal balanced: 30% low-glycemic carbohydrates, 30% unsaturated fats (preferably monounsaturated), 30% proteins, and 10% fruits every day. This diet will stimulate production of glucagons instead of insulin. Glucagons utilize fat, lower blood pressure, decreases triglycerides and LDL cholesterol, and raise HDL cholesterol. I recommend also an exercise program of walking for a half hour daily and stretch exercise for 5 to 10 minutes after walking. The short answer is yes.

Q. Is it true that eating fat makes you fat?

A. Of course not; lots of people think this despite the scientific basis for their wrongful reasoning. Fats are the last foods digested in a meal that is why they have a satiety value. One gram of fat gives almost as twice energy as much energy as one gram of protein or carbohydrate. Eating carbohydrate is the number one culprit in gaining weight because carbohydrates are easily converted into glucose for body use or storage as fat.

Q. How did ancient cultures treat obese bodies before the advent of the pharmaceutical companies and our modern medicine?

A. Howard Carter in A.D. 1922 found six dried bulbs of garlic in the 19- year- old king (Tutankhamen)Tot's tomb (buried more than five- thousand years ago). Cornflower, grape, groundsel, hyacinths, and yarrow were found also in Shindar, Iraq. Shindar is a prehistoric burial site for the Neanderthal species; a close relative to modern humans. The answer to your question is they used herbal medicine. Alfalfa has saponin that makes fats more soluble and the leaves contain flavones, isoflavones and sterols. Seaweed (kelp- agar) strengthens the thyroid, which increases the rate of metabolism. Cardamom has soothing and antispasmodic properties in the digestive tract. Cinnamon creates a thermogenic burn, reduces cholesterol (LDL) and leaves HDL unchanged. Actually, cinnamon is very effective in drinks or foods as anti-obesity agent. Fennel (*Foeniculum vulgare*) reduces hunger and improves energy. Use one teaspoon fennel seed in a cup of boiling water. Flax seed is a bulk laxative that helps curb hunger and is loaded with vitamins and polynutrients. Flax seeds taken an hour before meals will help you eat less, so you will lose weight while simultaneously strengthening your immune system. Parsley curbs appetite and reduces hunger cravings. Actually, carrot and parsley juices can help maintain proper blood sugar levels, and reduce blood sugar swings that you experience when on a weight loss program. *Phsyllium* helps to curb hunger and allows the elimination of waste from the body. It's effective because of the spongy fiber (mucilage) in the seeds and to specific chemicals (polyphenols) in the leaves. A teaspoon of phsyllium in water 30 minutes before meals reduces body weight significantly over time. Red pepper (*Capsicum spp*) and mustard raise metabolic rate as much as 25%. These hot spices also stimulate thirst, so you drink more liquids that also help in gaining less weight. *Citrus aurantium* (Chinese herb) is as effective as Ephedra in increasing thermo genesis in the body without the side effects that often result with the use of ephedra. *Citrus aurantium* or Zhi Shi contains a combination of adrenergic amines. These are synephrine, N-methyltyramine, hordenine, octopamine, and tyramine; they are powerful thermogenic agents. Eat *Citrus aurantium* fresh daily. Finally, garlic has been used to treat asthma, parasite infection, hemorrhoids, kidney stones, and menstrual abnormalities. It also lowers fat and cholesterol levels in blood. Garlic thins the blood, which helps to prevent clots inside the blood vessels, and thus may reduce the risk of heart attacks and strokes. Allin, a sulfur-containing amino acid in garlic, helps to boost the levels of HDL because it delivers excess cholesterol to the liver to be destroyed and simultaneously slows down endogenous cholesterol synthesis. Garlic is a terrific "cholesterol buster." 500 milligrams three times a day are recommended for healthier living. There are few side effects of garlic consumption, such as body odor, bad breath, heartburn, and flatulence. To overcome odor problems, wrap the clove in a peppermint leave and swallow it whole. Be sure to add the garlic at the end of cooking because the main ingredient "allin" vaporizes into air by cooking.

Q. I am taking allergy shots; is it possible to stay away from allergy medications if I eat right?

A. Most allergies are caused by food (allergens). Try to eliminate one food at a time from your diet to determine which food is causing the allergy. Mostly, gluten (in wheat) and casein in milk products are the major allergens. Otherwise, something in water or air is causing the allergy. Try it by elimination. For example, substitute milk with soy or rice milk, and stay away from casein sources in packaged foods, butter, cocoa butter, cream of Tartar, and calcium lactate. There is gluten- free bread available in some specialty stores.

Q. Do any sugar-coated pills or gums cause significant insulin surge?

A. No, because the sugar coating in pills or gums are usually in a very small amount.

Q. How much exercise is enough for a good health?

A. That depends upon your age and profession. Walking one mile a day is usually enough; it burns about 100 calories. Actually, I recommend a half-hour of walking every day and five to ten minutes of stretch exercise after walking.

Q. What is a portion or serving?

A. Based on the Food Pyramid serving's recommendations portion is one medium apple, peach, nectarine, two small plums, or medium size potato. It is a fistful -size food.

Q. Do I have to take supplement pills to complement my healthy diet?

A. Supplement pills are not necessary for three major reasons: a) your body is clever enough to scavenge all trace elements and vitamins needed. b) Most supplements have the active and the non-active forms of the needed vitamin; vitamins E and D are the best examples. c) Risk of overdose is greater than the benefit of supplementation. All supplements are in natural fruits and vegetables; eat fresh fruits and vegetables. Humankind lived, championed the Neolithic Revolution, and built the Great Pyramids in Giza, Egypt, created arts, languages, religion, architecture, sciences and medicine, and knowledge for six-thousand years without supplemental pills of nowadays. Eat natural, whole food.

Q. What are your thoughts about Olestra and likes as weight-loss supplements?

A. Olestra sucks away fat-soluble vitamins like A, D, E, and K.; especially vitamin A. Olestra is not a fat; it is a sucrose polyester. Ephedra helped people to lose weight, but put people at risk of heart attacks. Chitosan is an extract from the shells of shellfish. They claim that it leads to weight loss by blocking fat absorption, but studies have shown otherwise. Finally, Bitter Orange works like Ephedra with the same side effects as Ephedra, such as increasing heart rate and blood pressure. In a nut shell, most of all the supplements out there are not regulated by the FDA and safety should be a major issue.

Q. What fruit juice do you recommend to lose weight?

A. Eating whole fruit is better than drinking fruit juice for many reasons: 1) you avoid the effect of chemicals and heat that were used during the extraction process. 2) You satisfy some of your daily requirement of fiber. 3) You avoid the sugar added during the extraction process. If you have to drink fruit juice for sickness or lack of teeth, drink unsweetened fruits.

Q. What is the effect of fasting on weight loss?

A. Fasting is practiced in different forms according to your faith. Some faiths abstain from eating certain foods for a month like in Christianity, and other faiths abstain from eating anything or having sex from dawn to sunset for a month; however, they are free to eat any food and have sex between sunset and dawn like in Islam. In either case, fasting is okay as long as faithful individuals do not indulge in eating everything after breaking their fast. Actually, God's (Allah in Arabic) moral lesson of fasting is an exercise for self -control and willpower. If you can abstain from eating certain foods or for certain times from eating or having sex for a month, you are equipped with the patience and willpower to conquer all your problems, such as obesity, high cholesterol, hypertension or diabetes. And the biggest lessons are feeling the pain of others for lack of food or

187

sex for whatever reason: sickness, poverty etc., and teaching us compassion. Before the advent of the Abrahamic Holy Scriptures' (Old Testament, New Testament and the Qur'an) recommendations of fasting (the Old Testament in 1,400 B.C., the New Testament in A.D. 41, and the Qur'an in A.D. 611,) humans had practiced fasting in different forms for tens of thousands of years and worshipped one God (Allah in Arabic) in different ways. The Great Pyramids of Giza (built almost 5,000 years ago) are recognition of the concept of life after death for those who live righteously and do well for others on earth; it's as the concept of heaven (joining loved ones, banquets and wedding feasts) or hell (torments) as Jesus Christ says in Mathew 5:20, "For I say to you, that unless your <u>righteousness exceeds</u> the righteousness of the scribes and Pharisees, <u>you will by no means enter the kingdom of heaven</u>." Basically, righteousness is a prerequisite for the kingdom of heaven.

Q. I love chocolate; where can I find good quality chocolate to complement my healthy diet?

A. Any chocolate with more than 70% cocoa is good and healthy. Valvrona and Le Noir American chocolate are two good brands of chocolate and are usually found in specialty stores.

Q. How much bread can I eat and stay on weight- loss diet?

A. One slice of bran bread has 20 grams of carbohydrates (80 calories) and has 110 calories in total. Since your total daily calorie allowance is 1,800- 2,000, two slices of bread will give you 220 calories; 160 calories of them are carbohydrates. Eating 1-2 slices of whole-grain or bran bread daily is about right. Oat bran is better because it only has 15 grams of carbohydrates and a total of 85 calories per slice.

Q. I like to drink beer, how many beers can I drink and still lose weight?

A. That depends upon other parts of your diet. Generally one can of beer (12 fluid ounces) have about 120 calories. Beer is composed of fructose (a low –glycemic- index carbohydrate). Just one to two beers a day are okay (about 250 calories) of your 2,000 calories daily allowance.

Q. I am taking a blood thinner, which food would you recommend cutting down?

A. Vitamin K is the major player in blood thinning. Vitamin K - rich foods such as spinach and broccoli have a clotting effect on blood. Maintain a healthy level of vitamin K- rich foods. Saturated and polyunsaturated fatty acids increase blood clotting; a ratio of polyunsaturated to saturated fatty acids greater than 0.8 is associated with increased blood clotting. Hence, substituting polyunsaturated fat for saturated fat reduces LDL cholesterol levels but may increase blood clotting. Fish oils (omega-3 fatty acids) decrease blood clotting and improve blood viscosity. Fish oils, in a dosage of 10 gram per day, have almost the same effect as 325 mg of Aspirin daily. **Note: Avoid taking continuously Aspirin for more than ten days because it may cause bleeding.**

Q. What is the difference between whole -wheat and whole-grain bread?

A. Whole- grain bread contains other grains other than wheat, such as oats and rye. As I explained in a previous question, they differ in their total calorie as well as their carbohydrate content. Remember, the coarser the bread, the better because it will slow gastric emptying, slow digestion and gives you the fiber needed to suck all those oxidants in your diet.

Q. Which snacks do you recommend for weight-loss?

A. Choose low -glycemic fruits such as apples, pears, or grapefruits. Stay away from high-glycemic fruits such as dates, ripe banana, and of course sweet oranges.

Q. I am pregnant, how many calories should I take daily to maintain a normal weight?

A. 500 calories more is required than for a non- pregnant woman. Daily allowances during pregnancy are 2,500 calories, lots of folic acid and iron- rich vegetables and fruits.

Q. What is the best oil for cooking?

A. Olive oil with burning point 420^0 F, grape-seed oil 420^0 F, peanut oil 450^0 F, and sesame oil 450^0 F are best for oven-cooked meals at temperature higher than 350^0 F (moderate oven temperature). However, unrefined canola oil 225^0 F, extra-virgin oil 320^0 F, and unrefined sunflower oil 225^0 F are suitable for cooking at lower temperatures.

Q. Is semolina flour okay?

A. Yes, it is because it is the remaining flour after the white component has been removed. Stay away from highly processed, fine flours.

Q. I was diagnosed with AIDS, should I stop breastfeeding?

A. A sound decision to make because breastfeeding transmits AIDS virus, hepatitis and other agents. Generally, women with a compromised immune system should not breastfeed. Healthy mothers' breast feeding combats occurrences of breast cancer. Breast cancer originally was coined nuns' disease, but advent of birth control pills and infrequent pregnancy caused the advent of breast cancer because of fluctuations of progesterone and estrogen, which cause mutations e.g. breast cancer cells. Birth control pills contain high levels of those breast cancers – causing hormones.

Q. What is the effect of microwave on food?

A. Microwave should only be used for heating food, not cooking. Children should be kept away from microwave because their bodies are still dividing and adults should stay away from microwave transmit ions too. Most appliance use 60 Hz power in the United States (50 Hz elsewhere). Microwaves are light waves; they travel in straight lines. so stay away from the microwave slits. In a Turkish study, cooking of pepper, pea, and broccoli in microwave affected their antioxidant activity, but not spinach. In sum, the type of vegetable is more important than the type of cooking e.g., microwave cooking. Generally, all vitamin C- containing foods should not be cooked in a microwave because vitamin C is destroyed by heat.

Q. How do high altitudes affect cooking?

A. At sea level, water boils at 212^0 F; with each 500- feet increase in elevation, the boiling of water is lowered by about 1^0 F. This decreased boiling point (due to decreased pressure) affects food preparation in two ways: 1) Water and other liquids evaporate faster and boil at lower temperature. 2) Leavening gases in breads and cakes expand more. High altitude areas are also prone to low humidity, which can cause the moisture in foods to evaporate quicker during cooking. Covering foods during cooking at high altitude helps to hold moisture. Cooking meat and poultry by simmering or braising methods may take up to one-fourth more cooking time when cooked at 5,000 feet above sea level. The pressure in the canner must be increased by 1 pound of pressure for each 2,000 feet elevation above sea level.

Q. *What are the causes of bad breath?*

A. There are many causes for bad breath (halitosis); among them are bacteria in the mouth, stomach and intestinal disturbances; bowel sluggishness, sinus or tonsil infection, alcohol and tobacco use, and medical conditions such as diabetes, duodenal ulcers, gastro-esophageal reflux, hypoglycemia, kidney or liver malfunction, and respiratory infection. Dental problems such as periodontal disease, tooth abscess, crooked teeth and gum disease cause bad breath.

Q. *Is it true that alcoholism is a source of bad breath?*

A. Excessive (more than two drinks a day) alcohol consumption causes digestive problems that lead to bad breath. Second, alcohol dries out the mouth, which reduces saliva production-saliva washes out and retards bacterial growth. Third, mouth washes with more than 25% alcohol have linked to an increased incidence of cancer. Try to use a mouth wash with little alcohol as possible and always rinse your mouth with water after gargling with the mouth wash.

Q. *What foods cause bad breath?*

A. Acidic foods creates environment for bacterial growth; high - fat and high-protein foods may not digest and give off gas. Some people have a hard time digesting meat and dairy products like senior citizens and eastern Jews (due to lactose intolerance), which result in bad breath. Sugar foods; garlic, onion and curry; blue cheeses, Camembert and Roquefort; fish, especially tuna and anchovies; acidic beverages such as coffee and tea; deficiency of vitamins B and C; and finally deficiency of zinc.

Q. What is effect of ozone in bottled water?

A. FDA and EPA consider concentrations of 0.1- 0.4 mg/ Liter of ozone are safe. Residual (excess) ozone is dangerous. State and federal agencies monitor bottle- water treatments in the United States. I do recommend filtration better than bottling; it is an economical and much safer method.

Q. Which is better treatment of water, distillation or filtration?

A. Distillation removes heavy metals and kills *E. coli* forms but concentrates volatile chemicals. Filtration removes heavy and organic substances but partially removes *E. coli* forms. I recommend both, distillation followed by filtration.

Q. Which couscous would you recommend?

A. I do recommend whole-wheat couscous.

Q. Which foods have caffeine?

A. Caffeine is found in coffee (mainly), tea, and cola soda; decaffeinated coffee or black or green tea is better.

Q. Are protein-rich dieters more prone to cancer than others?

A. Protein - rich diets make body fluids more acidic and cancer cells favor acidic conditions. Therefore, fresh fruits and vegetables are recommended to accompany steak and grilled-chicken dishes.

Q. What is the right balance between harmful and beneficial time of exposure to sunlight?

A. 15- 20 minutes of daily exposure to sunlight are enough to satisfy our needs of vitamin D especially between 10 a.m. and 4 p.m.

Q. Does tanning satisfy our needs of vitamin D?

A. Not really, because tanning causes melanin to protect the body from burning. It is the production of melanin that causes the skin to darken and produce the tan. Tanning beds do not cover all light spectrum needed for production of vitamin D as sun lights do. Keep teenagers away from tanning beds and sunlamps. Walking in sunlight for 20 minutes helps in many ways: get your dose of vitamin D, regulate your blood pressure, and most importantly to lose weight. Walking has a psychological pump to your self-esteem too.

Q. How can I prevent "raccoon eyes?"

A. Although lifting eye- wear is never recommended during a tanning session, occasional adjustment is advisable to a new position to prevent raccoon eyes. Contact lenses are not recommended during tanning sessions because tanning draws moisture from eyes and contact lenses sometimes cause discomfort.

Q. What is the difference between yam and sweet- potato?

A. a 1/2 cup of cubed, raw yam has 21 grams of carbohydrates (84 calories), but a 1/2 cup of mashed sweet -potato has almost 40 grams of carbohydrates (160 calories).

Q. What diet do you recommend to control flatulence?

A. Generally, low insoluble-fiber diets are the best to control flatulence. Also sweeteners like sorbitol and mannitol are the worst offenders. Sulfur -rich foods such as eggs, beer, beans, cauliflower, and meat are also producers of hydrogen sulfide (the bad smell) upon digestion by intestinal bacteria. I need to emphasize that flatulence is a natural process. Actually, we usually produce about a liter of gas daily. Chewing gum, drinking carbonated drinks (soda), and smoking increase flatulence by increasing air intake. I just recall that non-flatulence was a major problem for the former president, Woodrow Wilson; he was relieved from his abdominal pain upon passing gases like we suppose to do; almost 10-12 passes a day.

Q. Are there any remedies to lessen flatulence?

A. Soaking beans a head of time is beneficial as well as eating lactobacillus-rich foods (certain yogurt and milk) - *Bifidus regularis-* reduces odor and eating leafy vegetables.

Q. *Is flatulence genetic or dietary?*

A. It is more dietary and pathogenic than genetic. In other words, some maladies such as colitis, celiac disease, irritable bowel syndrome, lactose intolerance, and spastic colon syndrome cause flatulence, as well as high insoluble- fiber diets.

Q. *Is coffee-mate okay?*

A. Coffee-mate (creamer) has 1 gram of fat (saturated) per tablespoon; use fat-free coffee mate because it is void of fat and has a low calorie content -10 calories per one tablespoon compared to 20 calories for the former coffee-mate.

Q. *What are the dietary treatments for high cholesterol?*

A. Total cholesterol of 200 mg/dl is desirable, 200-230 mg/dl is borderline, and 240 mg/dl or above is high cholesterol level. Your liver makes 70-90% of your body's daily cholesterol and the rest is obtained from dietary sources. Since your body gets approximately 20% of its daily requirements from dietary sources, a treatment strategy for high cholesterol has been to control cholesterol intake. Cholesterol is found in egg yolk, red meat, whole milk and organ meats (liver and brain). Fiber is known to bind dietary fat and cholesterol in the gut and thus inhibit their absorption by your body. Increasing your intake of green leafy vegetables has shown to have dramatic effects on blood cholesterol. There are several naturally occurring substances that have been known to significantly decrease blood cholesterol, such as garlic, niacin (vitamin B3), and Guggul. Guggul is an extract of the Indian herb (Commiphore mukul) and has no side effects.

Q. *Is it okay to eat Halloween's pumpkin seeds?*

A.85 pumpkin seeds (1 ounce) have 127 calories (16 grams carbohydrates, and 5 grams of each of fat and protein) and no fiber.

Q. Which pickle process would you recommend for weight-loss foods?

A. Pickling is done with lots of sugar or salt to inhibit bacterial growth. Neither salt nor sugar is good for a healthy diet because high salt causes high blood pressure and high sugar causes insulin surge. Heat-sterilized pickling is better; without sugar or salt addition.

Q. *Is there any danger of eating game meat?*

A. Game meat especially deer (white -tail) can transmit very small organisms, prions. Prions are transmitted by saliva, blood and raw meat. Prions are implicated in scrape, Kuru, TME, and CJD diseases. I usually cook the meat thoroughly and throw away organ meat. Be sure to wear white socks and long boots for hunting to avoid Lyme disease. Lyme disease is transmitted by the tick deer and caused by the bacteria *Borrelia burgdorferi* that is transmitted to humans by ticks (mainly deer ticks). Here some very interesting finding about Lyme Disease: 1) the tick does no harm to your body if removed before 24 hours of infestation because the tick takes time to attach itself to your body to suck your blood and transmit the diseases- moral lesson: take shower after hunting and remove all tick infestations; 2) there are many strains of the bacteria and therefore multiple drugs are needed to combat infection; and 3) avoidance of tick infestation is far better remedy for Lyme Disease than treatment.

Q. *Is there any danger from using sweeteners?*

A. In PKU (Phenylketonuria), phenylalanine (an essential amino acid) is not converted into tyrosine; aspartame (sweetener) contains phenyalanine and its consumption should be restricted in PKU patients especially children. Other problems are flatulence and diarrhea. Furthermore, they do not help in weight loss.

Q. *A friend gave me a tea plant. Is tea (green tea) produced from a specific plant and does black tea have the same benefits?*

A. There are many species of the genus *Camellia*; however, tea is produced from *Camellia sinensis* only. Green tea is the unfermented leaf of the tea leaf. Black tea is produced by piling up the leaves in heaps and briefly "sweated," a natural fermentation process that darkens the leaves and gives them their flavor and aroma. All tea forms contain theophylline; a close relative of caffeine and a natural stimulant. Green tea has EGCG, and in combination with tamoxifen, is effective in suppressing breast cancer *in vivo* and *in vitro*. Green tea also raises metabolic rates and speeds up fat oxidation; cholesterol is not a fat but a sterol. Green tea also relieves stress. According to a study in the J. of Psychopharmacology, 50 minutes after a high stress event, subjects who drank 4 cups of black tea per day for a 4 -week period experienced an average cortisol drop of 47%, compared to 27% for the placebo group- cortisol is a stress hormone. A cup of green tea- contains between 15 and 50 milligrams of caffeine- can help stop excess iron damaging to the bodies of people who suffer from haemochromatosis and Parkinson's disease because of its high content of tannin which limits iron absorption. The side effects of drinking tea are fluoride toxicity and caffeine addiction. Interestingly, adding milk to tea will block the normal, healthful effects that tea has against cardiovascular diseases; however, soy milk, does not contain casein and not known to have similar effects on tea. Green unroasted coffee beans decrease sugar absorption and help in weight loss.

Q. *Is it okay to eat eggs if I have heart problems in my family?*

A. Egg yolk and organ meat are the worst enemies for somebody like you because they are full of cholesterol. For example, one large egg has 213 milligram of cholesterol in yolk and zero milligram of cholesterol in the white part. I advise eating only the white part. Organ meat like liver and brain are other non-desirable foods for people with history of heart disease. Cook the white part in canola oil to get the necessary omega-3 fatty acids.

Q. *during a doctor's visit, I had a bone density test and I am thinking about Hormone Replacement Therapy (HRT). What are your thoughts on RHT?*

A. In 1997, several studies followed women who took estrogen replacement therapy (HRT) for more than five to ten years. They found a 40% increase in breast cancer, significant decrease in LDL (bad cholesterol), significant increase of HDL (good cholesterol), and a tremendous increase in C-reactive proteins. C-Reactive proteins are the major culprits of the inflammation in the artery. It is a much predictor of future heart attacks than cholesterol, especially in women. Further, HRT patients suffered the risk of developing blood clots in the legs and gallbladder disease. Other studies of Estrogen/Progestin Replacement Therapy (HERS) showed an increase of heart attacks, especially in the first year. The bottom line: 1) wait for your bone density test results and follow your physician's advice; 2) eat calcium -rich diet and use a weight-bearing exercise program (walking). Calcium is found in fortified (A& D) milk and green leafy vegetables. Calcium absorption occurs only in presence of vitamin D. Exposure to sunlight for 20 minutes daily provides our needs of vitamin D.

Q. What are the major factors that affect cholesterol levels?

A. Your cholesterol levels depend on several factors. Diet: saturated, cholesterol -rich, and polyunsaturated fat intake increase cholesterol levels. Exercise: regular walking for a 1/2 hour and 5-10 minutes of exercise after walking decrease cholesterol levels. Exercise lowers LDL levels and raises HDL cholesterol levels. Heredity: high blood cholesterol levels are inherited 30%; in other words, 3 out of ten with high cholesterol levels inherited their high cholesterol from their parents. Weight: over-weight and obesity are usually correlated with high cholesterol levels. Losing weight can help lower LDL cholesterol and total cholesterol levels, as well as increase HDL cholesterol. Age and gender: as you get older, cholesterol levels rise. Before menopause, women tend to have lower total cholesterol levels than men of the same age. After menopause, however, women's LDL levels tend to rise. Finally, certain medications and medical conditions can cause high cholesterol.

Q. How come we have the highest percentage of obese people although we work harder and we are more affluent than any other nation?

A. Obesity in our country is a result of many factors such as stress and wrong diet. The Mediterranean diet (the best diet in the world) is full of monounsaturated fats such as olive oil and canola oil. However, our western diet (the worst diet in the world) is full of saturated and polyunsaturated fats as in butter, margarine, and whole milk; and lacks the essential omega-3 fatty acids. The Mediterranean diet "antioxidant diet " includes up to 20% of total calories from fat (largely monounsaturated fat and omega-3 fats) and generous amounts of dietary antioxidants from plant sources that decrease the overall mortality and morbidity. Stress is a main factor, in our society, because we have to worry about basic necessities of life like healthcare, housing, employment, and education. This does not mean that I am in favor of socialism. Let me tell what John Kenneth Galbraith once quipped, "Under capitalism man exploits man. Under communism, it's just the opposite." Or the American Novelist, Norman Rush said, "Capitalism and socialism both have their contradictions, and it may turn out that socialism's contradictions just happened to be fatal first." It's very hard to think the young lad, Neil Ibrahim, at The George Washington University, honor student and excellent employee at a Washington, D.C. law firm at the same time at age 16 not a capitalist. Capitalism is more than a slogan, it's a competition with risk of <u>capital</u>, <u>time</u>, and <u>expertise</u> to make a <u>profit</u>; e.g. partnership in a Law firm is capitalism, but salaried employees are not capitalists because they are guaranteed salaries in exchange for their expertise without any risk of capital. The key words in capitalism are <u>risk</u> of your own capital and <u>profit</u>.

Q. Are you against eating at fast foods?

A. Of course not; I just advise everybody to look at the menus and   watch for sodium, calorie, and fat content. Do not super size meals. Avoid side dishes and desserts because they are sometimes loaded with bad fats, more calories, and simple sugars than the main dishes. Choose low-calorie dressing, not low-fat. Low-fat dressings are steeped in HFCS, which has plenty of calories, and the simple sugar (fructose) tricks your body into staying hungry.

Q. What is the effect of a protein-rich diet on Gouty Arthritis?
Dietary advice consists of restricting overly excessive alcohol intake especially beer and mineral spirits, weight reduction, and a decline in purine- rich foods, such as red meat, lentil, beans, and seafood, and turkey. There is a potentially protective effect with consumption of dairy products. Gouty arthritis is caused by intense inflammation secondary to monosodium urate crystal deposition in joints, kidneys, and soft tissues that causes clinical manifestations. Factors that contribute to this deposition are changes in pH level (e.g., ketosis in surgical patients); lower body temperature- explaining nocturnal attacks; and the level of particular dehydration because of diuretic therapy. Elevated serum uric acid levels do not develop gout. Data show that the annual incidence of gout is 0.5 percent in persons with a uric acid level between 7 and 8.9 mg per deciliter (415 and 530 [micro] mol per L), and the annual incidence is 4.5 percent in those with a level of 9 mg per deciliter (535 [micro] mol per L) or greater. Gout arthritis most commonly begins with involvement of a single joint or multiple joints in the lower extremities, most commonly in the first at foot, ankle, or knee joints. Pain, redness (erythema), and swelling often begin in the early morning and increase and peak within 24 to 48 hours. The pain is severe, and patients often cannot wear socks or touch bed sheets during flare-ups. Even without treatment, the attacks typically subside within five to seven days. Gouty arthritis is usually treated with prescribed Allopurinol or Probenecid but Aspirin 400 to 600 mg/ daily and dietary therapies work well.

Q . What is the effect of diet on sleep?

Sleep is controlled (on/off) primarily by melatonin (a substance in the brain) and melatonin is controlled by light. To have a good quality sleep, you need to eat early (3-4 hours before bedtime) and avoid heavy liquid (water, liquor or soft drinks) intake before bedtime because the more you drink; the more you have to urinate, which interrupts sleep. Always go daily to bed at the same time with lights off, and as soon as you awake turn the lights on to synchronize your biological sleep clock daily. 8 hours of sleep time daily is normal for most adults, but 6-8 hours of sleep time is not an unusual for older people. Remember, dreams indicate good night of sleep; therefore, have sweet dreams, and most importantly, your body will always make up for lost hours of sleep by disorientation, lack of concentration, fatigue and excessive sleepiness in other times. If you could not have 8 hours of sleep in one night, stay awake until the usual time to go to bed to synchronize your body back to the usual sleep cycle. Finally, banana, turkey meat and tuna- rich meals induce sleeping, as well as blue and dim lights do too.

This is probably beyond your interest or knowledge, but here is the physiological importance of sleep: During sleep, cerebrospinal fluid (CSF) circulates into brain cells to wash out toxins and other residues from brain cells. This CSF's function is a energy –demanding process and only sleep can provide such energy-demanding process to proceed for two main reasons: 1) during sleep, brain cells shrink to allow CSF to fill all brain cells; and 2) during sleep, brain cells require less energy to maintain other functions of brain e.g., body maintenance and dreaming. By the way, this also explains the correlation between Alzheimer disease's beta Amyloidal proteins accumulation because of lack of sleep or insomnia.

Cognitive Behavioral Therapy (CBT) is the best treatment for the 15% of Americans, who have chronic insomnia. Chronic insomnia is the deprivation of full sleep time (6-8 hours/ day) for three months. CBT centers on lessening the deleterious thoughts (lack of concentration at work or feeling drowsy) about loss of sleep, and going to bed late to shorten deleterious thoughts of insomnia. Naps and biphasic sleep (division of sleep time into two periods during 24 hr period as common among Chinese workers) are not recommended to relieve insomnia; actually they may aggravate insomnia. Just remember you will sleep when you are the least anxious about lack of sleep, and your brain is devoid of bad thoughts and anxiety.

Chapter 20

You are on Deck

"No man resolved to make the most out of himself has time to waste on personal Contentions." Abraham Lincoln

Ibrahim is the name for the patriarch Abraham (in the Bible and the Qur'an) because Abraham is the English translation of Ibrahim at King James Bible in AD 1611 from Latin to English, and the patriarch Ibrahim was born in2167 B.C. in Ur (present-day Kuwait) in the Arabian Peninsula. The patriarch Abraham in English (Ibrahim in Arabic and Samarian) had **eight** sons from three wives: Ishmael from Hagar; Isaac from Sara (Abraham's half –sister; incest!) ten years later at her old age of 86 (miracle); and six sons from Keturah: Zimran, Jokshan, Medan, Midian, Ishbak, and Shuah,) Genesis 24 and 25, NKJ Study Bible, Nelson Publishing, Nashville, Ten, 1997). Translation of the Bible from Latin to English by a decree from King Henry VIII of England made the Bible available to the laity and weakened the hold of the church on people's life. The Vatican denied King Henry VIII's request to divorce his first wife because she did not bear him a son, and therefore he established the Angelical church (chasm of the Catholic church of Rome) and accused his first wife with adultery, which is treason for a queen and punishable by beheading just like customs of the time in the Roman Empire (crucifixion was reserved for non-Roman citizens under Roman laws). To make the story short, King Henry VIII put to death five wives for treason for the sake of a son to inherit the throne of England; sadly his only son, Edward, died at age 15, and his daughter was the first female to inherit the throne of England after his death. Polygamy is sanctioned and practiced in the Bible from Moses, David, to others, and the Qur'an sanctions polygamy as well as our US Constitution does not mention or deal with marriage or polygamy despite our forefathers' awareness of marriage importance because they were married with kids. Marriage and other personal issues were left for the tenth amendment of the US Constitution or in other words under states' jurisdiction.

In baseball game," Ibrahim on deck" means either Dean Ibrahim or I will be playing next. Dean played for VFW and I played for Southern Printing. Well done. Now it is your turn to be in charge of your own health and most of all help others to enjoy the same health like you. Here are some suggestions to put you in charge:

1) Make it a habit to weigh yourself, once a week, and record your body weight; most grocery stores have **free** scales.

2) Make it a habit to measure your blood pressure, once a week, and record your blood pressure; all grocery stores' pharmacies have **free** blood pressure measurements equipments.

3) Attend your hometown Public Water Board meeting each month and be informed about the level of contamination in your public water system.

4) Call EPAs Safe Drinking Water Hotline: 800-426-4791 to know about drinking water in your state.

5) Call Community-Right-to- Know Hotline: 800 424-9346 to know about chemicals in your state that might affect your water quality and air quality.

6) Attend parents' meeting in your school and assure that your child's meals are prepared and cooked healthy for your child, as well as for others in school.

7) Spread the word about healthy living, do some bragging about your success, and most of all help others to achieve their goals. It pays a lot of dividends to help others to achieve their goals. The golden rules of my mom come to mind," Never look down on others unless you are pulling them up to stand on their own."

Finally, I would like to close with some sweet words of Jesus Christ from the book of Mathew (NKJ Study Bible, 1997):

"Ye shall know them by their fruits. Do men gather grapes of thorns or figs of thistle? Even so, every good tree bringeth forth good fruit but a corrupt tree bringeth forth evil fruit wherefore by their fruits ye shall know them."

Layman's Glossary

AIDS (Acquired immunodeficiency syndrome) is caused by HIV (virus). Symptoms include fever or night sweats, coughing, sore throat, fatigue, body aches, weight loss, and enlarged lymph nodes.

Acupuncture: The insertion of a needle into a tissue for the purpose of drawing fluid to relieve pain. It is very common in ancient Chinese medicine to cure illnesses.

Adrenal glands: two glands located above each kidney.

Allergen is an antigen that evokes an allergic reaction.

Alzheimer's disease is a disabling, progressive neurological disorder characterized by dysfunction and death of neurons resulting in impairment of intellectual and behavioral abilities.

Amino acid: One of the twenty amino acids required to build up proteins.

Antigen A: Substance has the ability to cause an allergic reaction.

Antioxidants: Chemicals that accept an oxygen-free radical and inhibits the oxidation of unsaturated fatty acids -those are important to maintaining health. Foods containing vitamins A, C and E are antioxidants.

Arthritis is an Inflammation of a joint.

Asthma: An allergic reaction resulting in wheezing and difficult breathing.

Atherosclerosis: A process in which fatty substances are deposited in the walls of arteries in response to hypertension, carbon monoxide, or dietary cholesterol; it causes damage and formation of plaques that decreases the size of the arterial vessel.

Bariatric Surgery: A procedure for mild obese people, whose lives are in danger from obesity.

Bile: A secretion of the liver consisting of water, bile salts, bile pigment, cholesterol, and several ions; it emulsifies lipids prior to digestion.

Bleeding time: The time required for the cessation of bleeding from a small skin puncture; it ranges from 4 to 8 minutes.

Blood pressure (BP): A measure of the pressure in arteries during heart contract (systole) and heart rest (diastole), 115 /75 is a healthy range.

Calorie: The unit of heat energy required to raise 1 kilogram of water from 14 to 15⁰ C (1 degree Celsius); the kilocalorie (Kcal), used in nutrition, is equal to 1000 calories.

Carcinogen: Any substance that causes cancer. Examples are X rays, radiations from intense exposure to sunlight, or radioactive materials.

Carnivore: An animal that eats other animals, either alive or dead. Examples are humans, lions, hawks, and jackals.

Carotene: Antioxidant vitamin; yellow-orange pigment present in the epidermis of vegetables and fruits such as carrots; also termed beta-carotene. It is a precursor to vitamin A.

Chlamydia: Prevalent sexually transmitted disease; characterized by burning on urination and low back pain. It may spread to uterine in females.

Cholesterol: A compound belongs to a family of sterols. It is usually combined with fat when circulating in the bloodstream for distribution to cells as LDL (lousy cholesterol) or HDL (good cholesterol).

Complex carbohydrates are carbohydrates with more complex structure, such as starch, glycogen or cellulose.

Cortisol: A steroid hormone made from cholesterol and produced from the adrenal cortex (in the kidney) that provides resistance to stress, dampens inflammation, and depresses immune response.

Diabetes mellitus type I: (juvenile) Diabetes because of lack of insulin and the resulting elevated blood glucose (sugar) levels.

Diabetes mellitus type II (over 40) is the result of resistance of the cells to the action of insulin which leads to elevated good glucose (sugar) levels. It is also characterized by increased urine production, excessive thirst, and excessive eating.

Diverticulitis is an inflammation of diverticulum (a sac or pouch in the wall of colon).

Energy: The capacity to produce motion or heat (work).

Enzyme: A protein that acts as a catalyst to speed up the reaction.

Fever is an elevation in body temperature above normal temperature 37^0 C (98.6^0 F).

Gallstone: A solid mass, usually containing cholesterol, in the gallbladder.

Gastric emptying is the process or time required to empty food from the stomach.

Glucose: A simple sugar (monosaccharide) that plays a key role in metabolism.

Goiter: An enlargement of the thyroid gland (close to Adam's apple).

Glycemic index measures how rapidly a certain carbohydrate food is digested into glucose and how fast it causes the blood glucose (sugar) to rise.

Hormone: A chemical compound that is secreted into the blood by a gland and that affects activities in other parts of the body.

Heartburn: Burning sensation in the esophagus because of reflux of acid from the stomach.

Hepatitis is the inflammation of the liver because of a virus, drugs, and chemicals.

HDL (high-density lipoprotein): Lipoproteins that carry cholesterol from the cells to the liver for breakdown and elimination from the body; it is the most determinant of risk for coronary artery diseases and heart attacks. HDL levels of more than 35 mg/dl are healthy.

Hiatus Hernia: A portion of the stomach protrudes to the esophagus.

Hyperglycemia: Abnormally elevated blood glucose (sugar) levels.

Hyperlipidemia: Abnormally elevated blood lipids, usually either cholesterol (LDL) or triglycerides or both.

Hypertension: Elevated blood pressure than 115/ 75 mm Hg.

Hypoglycemia: An abnormally low blood glucose (sugar) levels than can result from excess insulin, injected or secreted or starvation.

Hypothermia: Lowering of body temperature below 35^0 C (95^0 F).

Insulin is a hormone secreted by the alpha cells of the pancreas to regulate glucose levels in blood. It also causes the liver to convert excess glucose into glycogen for storage.

Insulin resistance is the failure of insulin to regulate glucose levels in blood, which causes elevated blood glucose levels and triggers the need for more insulin.

In vitro: Outside the body.

In vivo: Inside the body.

Lipase: An enzyme that digests fats and converts them into fatty acids and glycerol.

Lipid: An organic compound- composed of carbon, hydrogen and oxygen- that is usually insoluble in water; examples include triglycerides, steroids, fats and oils, cholesterol, and eicosanoids.

Lipogenesis is the formation of fat from glucose.

Lipolysis is the breakdown of triglycerides to free fatty acids and glycerol for energy use.

Lyme disease is a disease caused by the bacterium *Borrelia burgdorferi* that is transmitted to humans by ticks (mainly deer ticks) and is often characterized by a bull's eye rash. Symptoms include joint stiffness, fever and chills, headache, stiff neck, nausea, and lower back pain.

Monosaturated fatty acids: Those fats that have only one double bond, such as omega -3 fatty acids or omega-6 fatty acids. They are usually liquid at room temperature and common in olive and canola oils.

Night blindness: Poor or no vision in dim light or at night although good vision is present during bright illumination; often caused by a deficiency of vitamin A or nocturnal hypotension.

Neurotransmitter: A chemical produced by a neuron.

Omentum: storage of fat around the stomach.

Pancreas A soft, oblong organ lying along the stomach.

Parts per Million (PPM): Milligram per liter (mg/l), is one part per million. Just like one minute in 2 years or a single penny in $10,000.

pH: A unit to express alkalinity (pH higher than 7), neutrality (pH =7) or acidity (pH lower than 7).

Placebo: A fake medication (just water) as a control.

Plaque A: Cholesterol-containing mass in the arteries. It is a mass of bacterial cells, dextrin (polysaccharide), and other debris that adheres to teeth.

Polyunsaturated fats: Those fats with two or more double bonds; most vegetable oils are polyunsaturated. They are usually liquid at room temperature. They are found in corn oil, safflower, and cottonseed oil.

Prions: Infectious agents that cause slow diseases in humans, sheep and other animals e.g., kuru.

Rickets: Condition affecting children because of a vitamin D deficiency.

Saturated fatty acids: Those fats with fully hydrogenated carbon atoms, such as most animal fats. They are usually solid at room temperature.

Sclera (e): The white coat that covers part of the eyeball.

Simple sugars (monosaccharide) are sugars like glucose (our body's fuel), fructose (fruit sugar, syrup, and beer), and galactose (milk sugar).

Syndrome X: the combination of insulin resistance, elevated insulin levels, elevated triglycerides, and hypertension.

Teratology: Study of abnormal development & inborn diseases.

Thermo genesis: The rate at which calories are burned

Tubal Ligation: A sterilization procedure in which the uterine tubes are tied and cut to prevent pregnancy.

Tuberculosis an infection of the lungs caused by the bacterium *Mycobacterium tuberculosis*; results in destruction of the lung tissues.

Vagus nerve (X): one of the twelve cranial nerves; severing this nerve in the upper body interferes with swallowing, paralyzes vocal cords and interrupts sensation from many organs including the stomach.

Appendix

Cooking Terms

Bake: Cooked in an oven uncovered unless the recipe calls otherwise; preheat the oven to the temperature given in the recipe- unless the recipe specifies otherwise.

Baste: Brush or spoon a glaze, a sauce, or drippings on food as it cooks to add flavor and to help the surface moist.

Beat: Use a brisk up- and-over with a spoon or whisk to add air to a mixture and make it smooth. Or use an electric mixer or rotary beater to achieve similar results.

Blanch: Briefly boil or steam a food to prevent spoilage during freezing, or to loosen skins for peeling.

Blend: To combine ingredients well, usually with a spoon or a mixer.

Boil: Cook in a rapidly bubbling water.

Braise: Quickly brown in hot skillet with a little oil; then cook slowly with a small amount of liquid in a covered pan on the top of the stove or in the oven.

Chill: Refrigerate to reduce the temperature of food.

Chop: Cut into small pieces.

Cool: Let stand at room temperature (75^0 F) to reduce temperature of the food. When a recipe call for "cool quickly," the food should be refrigerated or set in a bowl of ice water to quickly reduce its temperature.

Cream: Beat with a spoon or a mixer to make mixture light and fluffy.

Dice: Cut into small cubes.

Dissolve: Stir a dry ingredient into a liquid until the dry ingredient is no longer visible.

Fillet: Cut from bone into serving portions.

Flake: Gently break into small pieces.

Fold: Gently combine two or more ingredients with an up-and-over motion with a spoon, whisk, or rubber spatula.

Fry: Cook in small amount of hot oil. When a large amount of oil is used, the process is called deep-fat (oil) frying.

Garnish: Add a decorative touch to food.

Glaze: Brush mixture on a food to give it a glassy appearance or a hard finish; usually the glaze adds a flavor to the food.

Grill: Cook on greased fry or griddle.

Grind: Use a food grinder to cut food into very fine pieces.

Knead: Work dough with the hands in a pressing, folding, and turning motion.

Marinate: Allow food to stand in a marinated liquid to add flavor or to make it much tender.

Mince: Cut into very tiny pieces.

Mix: Combine or blend ingredients.

Pare or peel: Strip off outer coating.

Partially set: A term used to describe gelatin mixture at the point in setting when the consistency resembles raw egg whites.

Pit: Remove the seed from a piece of fruit.

Poach: Cook in barely simmering liquid, being careful that the food holds its shape.

Puree: Use a blender, food processor, food mill, or potato masher to convert a food into a liquid or a heavy paste.

Reduce: Boil rapidly to evaporate liquid till mixture becomes thicker.

Roast: Cook meat, uncovered, in oven. "Pot roasting" refers to braising a meat roast.

Sauté: Cook, uncovered, in a small amount of oil over medium-high heat.

Scald: Bring to a temperature just below boiling so that tiny bubbles form at the edges of the pan; it also means to pour boiling water over food.

Score: Cut shallow gashes or slits through the outer layer of a food.

Sear: Brown surface of meat quickly with high heat.

Shred: To break or cut into thin pieces.

Sift: Pass flour or dry mixture through a sieve or a sifter to incorporate air and break up lumps.

Simmer: Cook in liquid that is just below the boiling point; bubbles usually burst before reaching surface.

Steam: Place food on a rack or a streamer gently above boiling water; cover with lid.

Steep: Extract the flavor or color from a food ingredient by letting it stand in a hot liquid.

Stew: Cook slowly in a simmering liquid.

Stir: To blend with a circular motion using a spoon until all ingredients are mixed well.

Stir-fry: Cook quickly in a small amount of hot oil with occasional stirring.

Toss: mix lightly with a fork or two forks.

Whip: To beat lightly and rapidly with a beater, incorporating air into a mixture to make it light and to increase its volume.

Oven Temperature Conversion Table

Temp	Fahrenheit (F)	Celsius (C)	Gas Setting
Warm	170	77	
	200	93	0-1/2
	225	107	
Very Low	250	221	1/2- 1
	275	135	
Low	300	149	1- 2
	325	163	
Moderate	350	177	2- 3
	375	191	4
Moderate Hot	400	204	5
Hot	425	218	6-7
	450	232	
Very Hot	475	246	8-9
	500	260	
	525	274	
Broil	550	288	

Metric Equivalents

Volume

Imperial	Metric
1/8 teaspoon	0.5 milliliter
1/4 teaspoon	1 milliliter
1 teaspoon	5 milliliters

1 tablespoon (1/2 fluid ounce) 15 milliliters^

1/4 cup (2 fluid ounces) 2 tablespoons (50 milliliters)

1 cup (8 fluid ounces)	1 cup (250 milliliters)
1 pint (16 fluid ounces)	500 milliliters
1 quart (32 fluid ounces)	1 liter minus 2 tablespoons

^ The Australian tablespoon is 20 milliliters, but the differences are usually negligible.

Cooking Points

Imperial	Metric
0^0 F	minus 19^0 C
32^0 F(water freezing point)*	0^0 C
180^0 F (water simmers)	82^0 C

212^0 F (Water boiling point)* 100^0 C

* Salt-free water, at sea level

Weight

Imperial	Metric
1/4 ounce	7 grams
1 ounce	28.4 grams
8 ounces (1/2 pound)	225 grams
35 ounces (2.2 pounds)	1 kilogram

1 table spoon= 3 teaspoons

1 cup= 1/2 pint= 16 tablespoons

1 pound= 16 ounces

Length

Imperial	Metric
1/2 inch	12 millimeters
1 inch	2.54 centimeters
12 inches (1 foot)	30 centimeters
1 mile (5280 feet)	1.61 kilometers

Measurements made using cups or spoons should be always leveled unless stated otherwise in recipes.

Food Ingredient Substitutions

Amaretti	Almond-flavored macaroons
Apple butter	Apple puree
Baking soda	Bicarbonate of soda
Butter crunch candy	Honeycomb
Cake flour	Sifted white flour
Cornstarch	Corn flour
Dragee	Sugared Almonds
Egg bread	Brioche
Flour, all -purpose	White flour
Graham crackers	Biscuits
Granola	Muesli
Jelly	Jam
Maple extract	Maple syrup
Mint extracts	Peppermint essence
Peppers (green, yellow or red)	Capsicums
Piecrust mix	Prepared or frozen pastry
Raisins, golden	Sultanas
Sugar, confectioners	icing sugar
Sugar, granulated	Ordinary white sugar
Sugar, superfine	Castor sugar
Vanilla extract	Vanilla essence

Fruits& Vegetables Rich in Vitamin C:

Banana, Cantaloupe, Grapefruits, Watermelon, Kiwi, Lemon (not lime), Oranges, Peaches, Pineapples, Strawberry and Tangerines

Fruits & Vegetables Rich in Vitamin A:

Carrots, Cantaloupe, Nectarine, Peaches, Tangerine, Broccoli, Green Onion, Sweet Potato and Tomato

Fruits & Vegetables Rich in Iron (to combat Restless Leg)**:**

Banana, Cantaloupe, Kiwi, Lime (not Lemon), Peaches, Sweet Potato, Sweet Corn, Strawberry, Broccoli, Green Cabbage, and Watermelons

Fruits & Vegetables Rich in Calcium (to combat Osteoporosis)**:**

Kiwi, Oranges, Grape Fruits, Sweet Potatoes, Broccoli, Green Lettuce and Green Cabbage

Recipes' Index

- The Index is meant to be numbered wrong to encourage you to go through all recipes.

Acknowledgments

I owe special thanks to many individuals and institutions that supported me in the course of Weight Loss' three – year gestation. I would like to thank Debbie Dyer and Stephen Lomax for their help with the water section; Jim Scott, owner of J & C Grocery, for providing the grocery for the calorie and content analyses; and JoAnn Green for her help with the computer search and of course Christa Simmons, M.S., my former LCHS classmate Engineer Kevan Vernon and Mrs. Genese Vernon for their computer expertise to make this book a reality. Last but not the least, I am grateful to my parents who advocate training one's self for a 1/3 of life, working for another 1/3, and help others in the last 1/3.

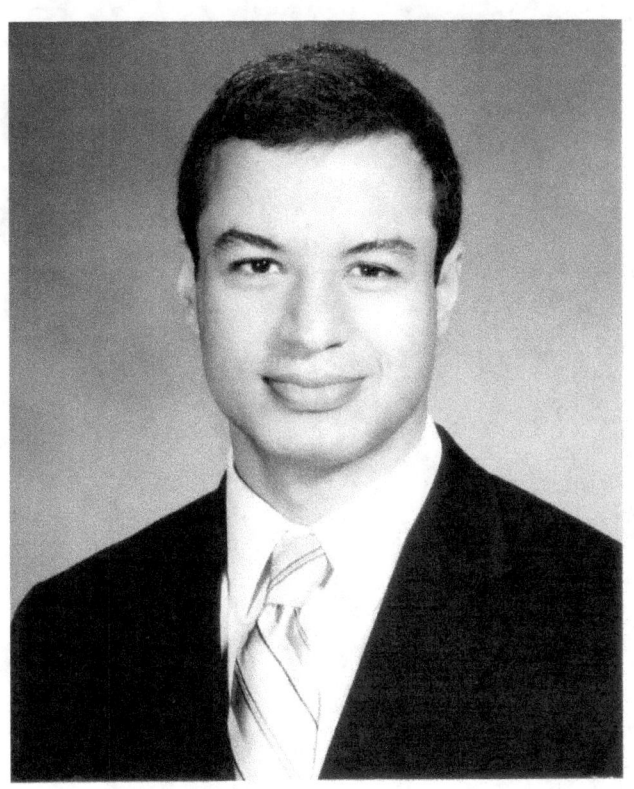

Neil Ibrahim, MD, the Texas native, is an alumnus of The George Washington University, Washington, D.C. and honor medical student; recipient of The George Washington University Alumni Award; and co-author of two more books with Dean Ibrahim, MD: ACT with Writing Option, and SAT II in Math II, Biology and Chemistry. He has/had been member of Sigma Nu fraternity of The George Washington University, Star at the Boy Scouts of America (BSA) in Lawrenceburg, Tennessee, and member of the American Medical Student Association (AMSA). He enjoys baseball, swimming, canoeing, as well as chess, basketball, hunting and horse-back riding during his leisure time in his estate in Tennessee, USA.

www.ingramcontent.com/pod-product-compliance
Lightning Source LLC
Chambersburg PA
CBHW060458290526
45791CB00001B/174